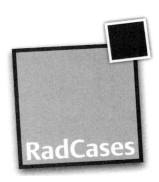

Pediatric Imaging

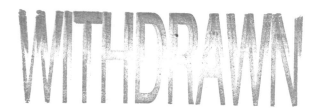

WITHDRAWN

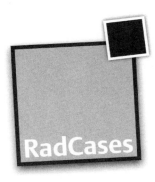

Pediatric Imaging

Edited by

Richard B. Gunderman, MD, PhD, MPH
Professor of Radiology, Pediatrics, and Medical Education
Vice Chair of Radiology
Department of Radiology
Indiana University School of Medicine
Riley Hospital for Children
Indianapolis, Indiana

Lisa R. Delaney, MD
Assistant Professor
Department of Radiology
Indiana University School of Medicine
Radiologist
Riley Hospital for Children
Indianapolis, Indiana

Series Editors

Jonathan Lorenz, MD
Associate Professor of Radiology
Department of Radiology
The University of Chicago
Chicago, Illinois

Hector Ferral, MD
Professor of Radiology
Section Chief, Interventional Radiology
RUSH University Medical Center, Chicago
Chicago, Illinois

Thieme
New York • Stuttgart

Thieme Medical Publishers, Inc.
333 Seventh Ave.
New York, NY 10001

Executive Editor: Timothy Hiscock
Editorial Director: Michael Wachinger
Editorial Assistant: Adriana di Giorgio
International Production Director: Andreas Schabert
Production Editor: Katy Whipple, Maryland Composition
Vice President, International Marketing and Sales: Cornelia Schulze
Chief Financial Officer: James W. Mitos
President: Brian D. Scanlan
Compositor: MPS Content Services
Printer: Sheridan Press

Library of Congress Cataloging-in-Publication Data

Pediatric imaging / edited by Richard Gunderman, Lisa R. Delaney.
    p. ; cm. — (RadCases)
  Includes bibliographical references.
  Summary: "Pediatric radiology is a special field. It is distinguished from most other radiologic disciplines by
the fact that it addresses all of the organ systems and imaging modalities. Moreover, it focuses on the most
formative and resilient stages of life, from infancy to adolescence. The patients it serves are in some respects
the most vulnerable and precious of all. Like other pediatric fields, it is populated by people of special optimism and dedication, and pediatric radiologists typically enjoy relationships of high mutual respect and
gratitude with patients, families, and referring health professionals. Studying pediatric radiology is a special
privilege, offering opportunities to explore the anatomy, physiology, and pathology of the developing human,
and to put to work for our patients some of the most remarkable diagnostic advances in the recent history
of medicine. We feel blessed to count ourselves among the long line of physicians who have practiced this
craft, and we offer these cases with the hope that they will enrich the quality of care of infants, children, and
adolescents for years to come"—Provided by publisher.
  ISBN 978-1-60406-181-9
  1. Pediatric radiology—Case studies. I. Gunderman, Richard B. II. Delaney, Lisa R. III. Series: RadCases
  [DNLM: 1. Diagnostic Imaging—Case Reports. 2. Child. 3. Infant. WN 240 P3713 2010]
  RJ51.R3P397 2010
  618.92'00757—dc22

                                                                                                    2010015026

Important note: Medical knowledge is ever-changing. As new research and clinical experience broaden our
knowledge, changes in treatment and drug therapy may be required. The authors and editors of the material
herein have consulted sources believed to be reliable in their efforts to provide information that is complete
and in accord with the standards accepted at the time of publication. However, in view of the possibility
of human error by the authors, editors, or publisher of the work herein or changes in medical knowledge,
neither the authors, editors, nor publisher, nor any other party who has been involved in the preparation of
this work, warrants that the information contained herein is in every respect accurate or complete, and they
are not responsible for any errors or omissions or for the results obtained from use of such information. Readers are encouraged to confirm the information contained herein with other sources. For example, readers are
advised to check the product information sheet included in the package of each drug they plan to administer
to be certain that the information contained in this publication is accurate and that changes have not been
made in the recommended dose or in the contraindications for administration. This recommendation is of
particular importance in connection with new or infrequently used drugs.

Some of the product names, patents, and registered designs referred to in this book are in fact registered
trademarks or proprietary names even though specific reference to this fact is not always made in the text.
Therefore, the appearance of a name without designation as proprietary is not to be construed as a represen-
tation by the publisher that it is in the public domain.

Printed in the United States

978-1-60406-181-9

For Laura, Rebecca, Peter, David, and John
—*Richard B. Gunderman*

For John, Lauren, Caroline, Lucas, and Evan
—*Lisa R. Delaney*

RadCases Series Preface

The ability to assimilate detailed information across the entire spectrum of radiology is the Holy Grail sought by those preparing for the American Board of Radiology examination. As enthusiastic partners in the Thieme RadCases Series who formerly took the examination, we understand the exhaustion and frustration shared by residents and the families of residents engaged in this quest. It has been our observation that despite ongoing efforts to improve Web-based interactive databases, residents still find themselves searching for material they can review while preparing for the radiology board examinations and remain frustrated by the fact that only a few printed guidebooks are available, which are limited in both format and image quality. Perhaps their greatest source of frustration is the inability to easily locate groups of cases across all subspecialties of radiology that are organized and tailored for their immediate study needs. Imagine being able to immediately access groups of high-quality cases to arrange study sessions, quickly extract and master information, and prepare for theme-based radiology conferences. Our goal in creating the RadCases Series was to combine the popularity and portability of printed books with the adaptability, exceptional quality, and interactive features of an electronic case-based format.

The intent of the printed book is to encourage repeated priming in the use of critical information by providing a portable group of exceptional core cases that the resident can master. The best way to determine the format for these cases was to ask residents from around the country to weigh in. Overwhelmingly, the residents said that they would prefer a concise, point-by-point presentation of the Essential Facts of each case in an easy-to-read, bulleted format. This approach is easy on exhausted eyes and provides a quick review of Pearls and Pitfalls as information is absorbed during repeated study sessions. We worked hard to choose cases that could be presented well in this format, recognizing the limitations inherent in reproducing high-quality images in print. Unlike the authors of other case-based radiology review books, we removed the guesswork by providing clear annotations and descriptions for all images. In our opinion, there is nothing worse than being unable to locate a subtle finding on a poorly reproduced image even after one knows the final diagnosis.

The electronic cases expand on the printed book and provide a comprehensive review of the entire subspecialty. Thousands of cases are strategically designed to increase the resident's knowledge by providing exposure to additional case examples—from basic to advanced—and by exploring "Aunt Minnie's," unusual diagnoses, and variability within a single diagnosis. The search engine gives the resident a fighting chance to find the Holy Grail by creating individualized, daily study lists that are not limited by factors such as a radiology subsection. For example, tailor today's study list to cases involving tuberculosis and include cases in every subspecialty and every system of the body. Or study only thoracic cases, including those with links to cardiology, nuclear medicine, and pediatrics. Or study only musculoskeletal cases. The choice is yours.

As enthusiastic partners in this project, we started small and, with the encouragement, talent, and guidance of Tim Hiscock at Thieme, continued to raise the bar in our effort to assist residents in tackling the daunting task of assimilating massive amounts of information. We are passionate about continuing this journey, hoping to expand the cases in our electronic series, adapt cases based on direct feedback from residents, and increase the features intended for board review and self-assessment. As the American Board of Radiology converts its certifying examinations to an electronic format, our series will be the one best suited to meet the needs of the next generation of overworked and exhausted residents in radiology.

Jonathan Lorenz, MD
Hector Ferral, MD
Chicago, IL

Preface

Pediatric radiology is a special field. It is distinguished from most other radiologic disciplines by the fact that it addresses all of the organ systems and imaging modalities. Moreover, it focuses on the most formative and resilient stages of life, from infancy to adolescence. The patients it serves are in some respects the most vulnerable and precious of all. Like other pediatric fields, it is populated by people of special optimism and dedication, and pediatric radiologists typically enjoy relationships of high mutual respect and gratitude with patients, families, and referring health professionals. Studying pediatric radiology is a special privilege, offering opportunities to explore the anatomy, physiology, and pathology of the developing human, and to put to work for our patients some of the most remarkable diagnostic advances in the recent history of medicine. We feel blessed to count ourselves among the long line of physicians who have practiced this craft, and we offer these cases with the hope that they will enrich the quality of care of infants, children, and adolescents for years to come.

Richard B. Gunderman, MD, PhD, MPH
Lisa R. Delaney, MD

Acknowledgments

A work of this nature reflects the contributions of many people. We wish to express our gratitude to the many medical students, diagnostic radiology residents, and pediatric radiology fellows with whom it has been our pleasure to learn. Thanks also to our current colleagues in pediatric radiology at Indiana University, including Mervyn Cohen, Donald Corea, Mary Edwards-Brown, Boaz Karmazyn, Francis Marshalleck, Molly Raske, Aslam Siddiqui, and Matthew Wanner, as well as former colleagues Kimberly Applegate, Eugene Klatte, and John Smith, from whom we have learned so much. We also thank John Krol for his help in compiling many of the cases, Ruth Patterson and Rhonda Gerding for cheerful secretarial support, and colleague Chang Ho for reviewing the neuroradiology cases. Above all, we offer our deepest thanks to our families for their patience and support as we labored over this project.

Case 1

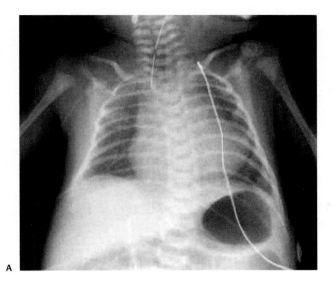

A

■ Clinical Presentation

....

Difficulty passing an orogastric tube in a neonate.

Further Work-up

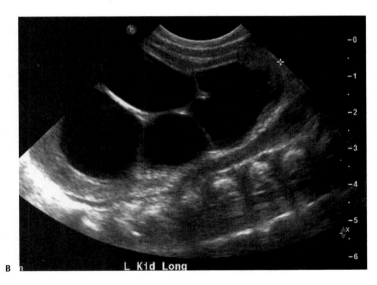

B

■ Imaging Findings

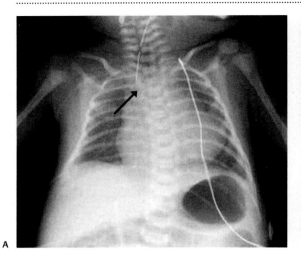 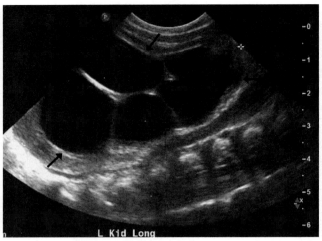

(A) Frontal chest radiograph demonstrates an esophageal tube with its tip in a proximal esophageal pouch (*arrow*), suggesting an esophageal atresia. The finding of gas in the stomach and bowel indicates an associated tracheoesophageal fistula. Cardiomegaly suggests congenital heart disease. **(B)** Longitudinal renal sonogram demonstrates multiple large renal cysts (*arrows*) that connect with the renal pelvis, consistent with severe hydronephrosis.

■ Differential Diagnosis

- **VACTERL association:** The combination of esophageal atresia/tracheoesophageal fistula and a congenital renal anomaly is highly suggestive of VACTERL association.
- *Esophageal perforation:* Placement of an esophageal tube can be complicated by perforation, but the lack of pneumomediastinum and/or pleural effusion argues against this, and tube malposition should not be associated with a renal anomaly.
- *Tracheal placement:* Placement of an esophageal tube into the trachea could have a similar appearance, but the proximal part of the esophagus should not be so dilated, and this would not be associated with a renal anomaly.

■ Essential Facts

- VACTERL is an acronym for a nonsyndromic constellation of findings that includes the following:
  - Vertebral anomalies—typically hypoplastic vertebrae or hemivertebrae
  - Anal atresia/imperforate anus
  - Cardiovascular anomalies—often an uncomplicated ventricular septal defect
  - Tracheoesophageal fistula
  - Renal anomalies, such as incomplete formation of one or both kidneys, obstruction of outflow of urine from the kidneys, or severe reflux
  - Limb defects often involving the radius and associated with absent or displaced thumbs and polydactyly/syndactyly

✓ Pearls & ✗ Pitfalls

- ✓ When limb defects are bilateral, renal involvement is usually bilateral; when the limb defect is unilateral, so typically are the renal defects.
- ✓ More commonly associated with maternal diabetes

Case 2

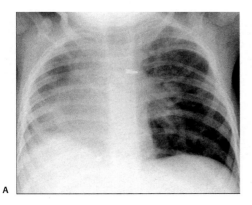

A

■ Clinical Presentation

A 2-year-old boy with chronic cough.

Further Work-up

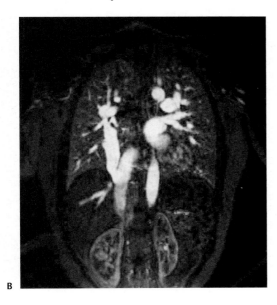

B

■ Imaging Findings

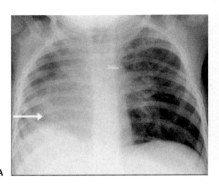
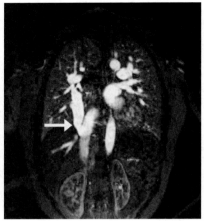

(A) Anteroposterior chest radiograph. There is a small right lung with shift of the heart and mediastinum to the right. Additionally, there is a curved opacity near the elevated right hemidiaphragm (*arrow*). **(B)** Coronal magnetic resonance (MR) image demonstrates an anomalous right pulmonary venous connection to the inferior vena cava (*arrow*).

■ Differential Diagnosis

- **Scimitar syndrome:** A hypoplastic right lung with visualization of an anomalous draining vein is consistent with scimitar syndrome.
- *Right lung hypoplasia:* No scimitar vein would be identified.
- *Pulmonary sequestration:* This appears as a mass in the right lung base with a relatively normal-size right lung. The arterial supply, but not necessarily the venous drainage, is systemic.

■ Essential Facts

- Right lung hypoplasia with anomalous right pulmonary venous connection to the inferior vena cava is also called *hypogenetic lung syndrome* or *congenital pulmonary venolobar syndrome.*
- It is often associated with absence of the right pulmonary artery and anomalous systemic arterial supply to the right lung.
- Signs, symptoms, and age at presentation are determined by the size of the shunt.
- Baffling of the pulmonary vein onto the left atrium is indicated when there is a large shunt.
- Chest radiograph shows right lung hypoplasia with a scimitar vein in the medial costophrenic sulcus, shunt vascularity.

■ Other Imaging Findings

- Computed tomography angiography or MR angiography can demonstrate the anomalous venous drainage and/or arterial supply.
- Conventional angiography is usually reserved for coil embolization if a systemic artery is identified.

✓ Pearls & ✗ Pitfalls

- ✓ *Scimitar sign* refers to the curved opacity near the right border of the heart that increases in diameter in the caudal direction, representing the anomalous vein.
- ✗ It can be difficult to distinguish from other anomalous pulmonary venous connections.

Case 3

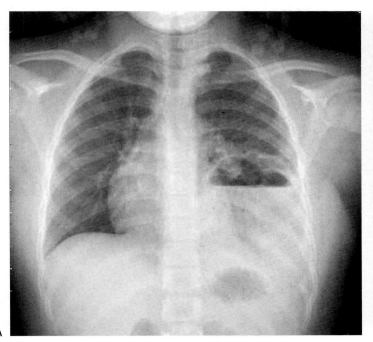

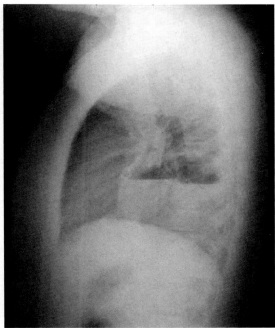

A

B

■ Clinical Presentation

A 10-year-old girl with recurrent pneumonia.

Further Work-up

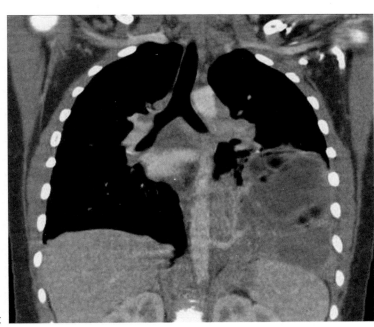

C

■ Imaging Findings

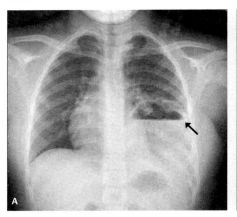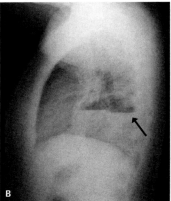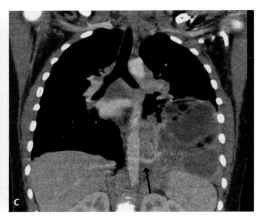

(A,B) Anteroposterior and lateral chest radiographs demonstrate a cystic mass in the left lower lobe with air-fluid levels (*arrows*). **(C)** Coronal post-contrast computed tomography image of the chest demonstrates a fluid-filled mass that contains air. Note the systemic blood supply arising from the descending aorta (*arrow*).

■ Differential Diagnosis

- *Pulmonary sequestration:* A lower lobe mass with a systemic blood supply is consistent with sequestration.
- *Congenital cystic adenomatous malformation (CCAM):* A cystic mass with air-fluid levels could represent CCAM; however, it would not have a systemic blood supply.
- *Bronchogenic cyst:* This is rarely multilocular and rarely contains air unless infected. The most common location is mediastinal rather than intrapulmonary, and it does not have a systemic blood supply.

■ Essential Facts

- A pulmonary sequestration is a congenital area of abnormal lung that does not communicate with the bronchial tree and has a systemic arterial supply.
- It most commonly presents as recurrent pneumonia.
- Treatment is resection in symptomatic cases; in asymptomatic cases, treatment is controversial.
- Two types that are very difficult to distinguish by imaging are the following:
  - Intralobar: This is located within a normal lobe, has no separate visceral pleura, and usually drains via pulmonary veins.
  - Extralobar: This develops as an accessory lung with its own pleura, usually has systemic venous drainage, and shows a 65% association with other anomalies.
- Persistent lung opacity is seen over multiple presentations.
- The condition is most common in the left lower lobe, then the right lower lobe.
- Systemic arterial supply most commonly arises from the descending aorta but may arise from below the hemidiaphragm; venous drainage varies.
- The sequestration typically does not contain air unless infected.

- Any modality that can identify the systemic artery feeding the sequestration can be used for diagnosis.

✓ Pearls & ✗ Pitfalls

- ✓ It does not appear as an air-containing mass in the neonatal period.
- ✓ Always consider sequestration in a patient with pneumonia that recurs in the same area.
- ✓ Diagnostic clincher: a systemic artery is feeding the mass.
- ✗ Extralobar sequestration may appear as a paraspinal mass and can be confused with neuroblastoma.

Case 4

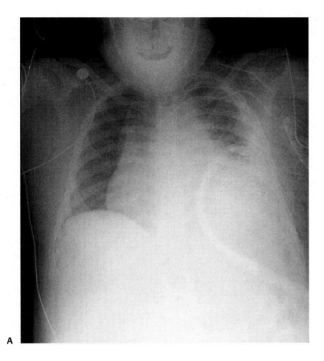

A

▦ Clinical Presentation

A 10-year-old boy with chest pain. A follow-up study was obtained after the acute episode.

Further Work-up

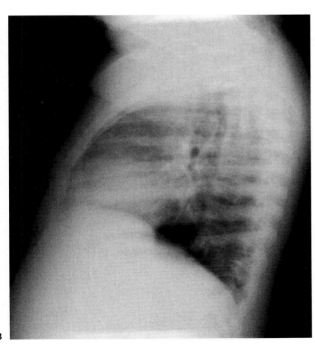

B

■ Imaging Findings

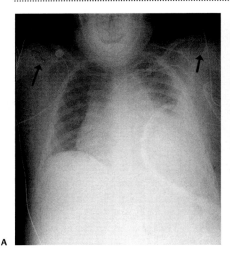 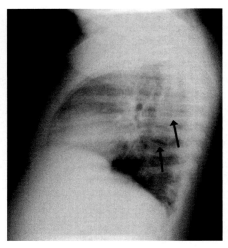

(A) Frontal chest radiograph demonstrates cardiomegaly and left lower lobe air space disease. There is irregularity of the humeral head epiphyses (*arrows*). (B) Lateral chest radiograph: there are multiple vertebral body end plate irregularities (*arrows*).

■ Differential Diagnosis

- ***Acute chest syndrome (ACS), sickle cell disease:*** The constellation of findings including cardiomegaly, humeral head and vertebral end plate changes, and air space disease points to ACS.
- *Community-acquired pneumonia:* Community-acquired pneumonia could have these chest radiograph findings, but it does not account for the bony and heart findings.
- *Aspiration pneumonia:* Aspiration pneumonia would have these chest radiograph findings, but it does not account for the bony and heart findings.

■ Essential Facts

- ACS is defined as the appearance of a new air space opacity accompanied by chest pain, leukocytosis, and fever in a patient with sickle cell disease.
- The exact cause of ACS is rarely determined, but it can be attributed to infection (30%), fat embolism, or rib infarction leading to splinting/atelectasis.
- ACS occurs in up to 50% of patients with sickle cell disease; the incidence is highest in children from 2 to 4 years of age.
- It is often recurrent and can lead to pulmonary hypertension and chronic lung disease.
- It is a significant cause of mortality in patients with sickle cell disease.
- Chest radiograph: Opacities may rapidly resolve; lower lobes predominate; cardiomegaly, pulmonary edema, and effusions are common; enlarged ribs arise from marrow expansion. Look for small, possibly calcified spleen and right upper quadrant cholecystectomy clips.

■ Other Imaging Findings

- Musculoskeletal plain films: findings include avascular necrosis of the humeral heads, H-shaped vertebral bodies, bony sclerosis because of infarcts.

✓ Pearls & ✗ Pitfalls

- ✓ Always look for bony changes, a splenic shadow, and gallstones or cholecystectomy clips in suspected cases of ACS.
- ✗ Because the exact etiology of ACS is multifactorial, it can have many radiographic appearances.

Case 5

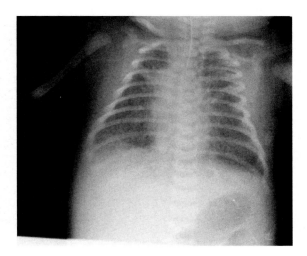

■ Clinical Presentation

A newborn infant with respiratory distress.

◼ Imaging Findings

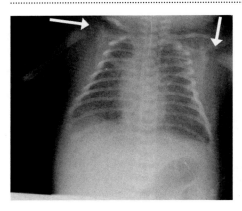

Frontal radiograph of the chest demonstrates coarse interstitial opacities with increased lung volumes. There is no pleural effusion. Notice that the humeral epiphyses are ossified (*arrows*), indicating that this is probably a full-term infant.

◼ Differential Diagnosis

- ***Meconium aspiration:*** Linear densities emanating from the hila and increased lung volumes are consistent with meconium aspiration.
- *Transient tachypnea of the newborn:* Although this also occurs in term infants, the course is benign, and intubation is not required. The diagnosis of transient tachypnea of the newborn may have pleural effusion.
- *Neonatal pneumonia:* This can also appear as asymmetric, patchy, perihilar densities with hyperinflated lungs. The diagnosis of neonatal pneumonia may have pleural effusion.

◼ Essential Facts

- Meconium aspiration most often occurs in term infants with in utero or intrapartum stress; it rarely occurs in infants born before 34 weeks' gestation.
- There is often a clinical history of meconium-stained amniotic fluid. Only meconium aspirated to below the vocal cords is clinically significant.
- Treatment includes immediate suction, then ventilation, antibiotics, surfactant, and inhaled nitrous oxide.
- Complications include pulmonary hypertension and those associated with mechanical ventilation: pneumothorax (20–40%), pneumomediastinum, pulmonary interstitial emphysema, and chronic lung disease.
- The severity of persistent pulmonary hypertension is a major prognostic determinant.
- The overall survival rate is 94%.
- Radiographic findings include increased lung volumes, heterogeneous opacities in the central two-thirds of lung, and frequent manifestations of air leak.
- The radiographic severity of disease does not correlate with clinical findings.
- The plain radiographic findings almost always return to normal by 1 year of age.

✓ Pearls & ✗ Pitfalls

- ✓ Meconium aspiration occurs in term infants.
- ✓ Pleural effusion is uncommon.
- ✗ It can appear identical to neonatal pneumonia—look for effusions to help differentiate.

Case 6

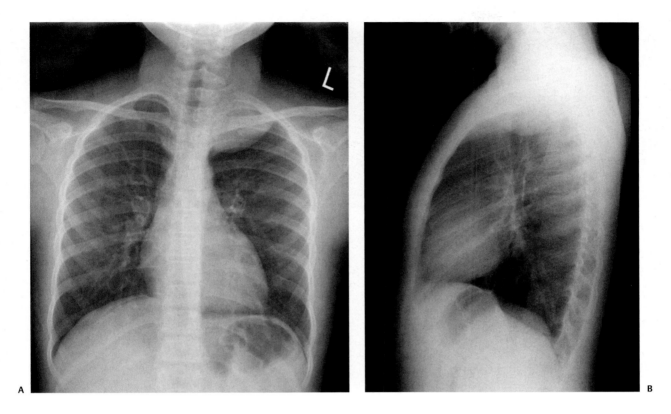

A

B

Clinical Presentation

A teenager with shortness of breath.

Further Work-up

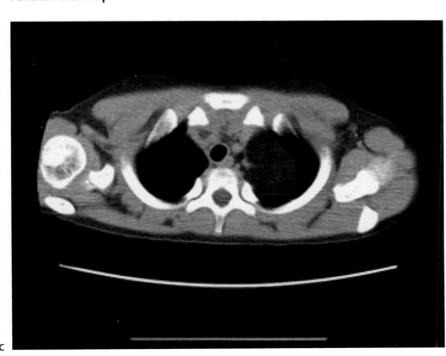

C

◼ Imaging Findings

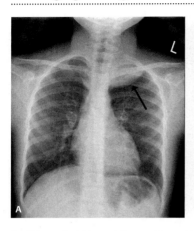 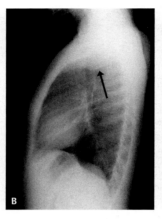 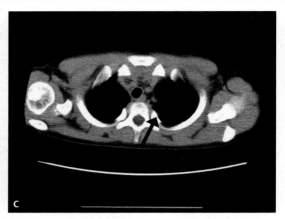

(A,B) Frontal and lateral chest radiographs demonstrate a smooth, well-defined soft-tissue mass in the apex of the left hemithorax (*arrows*). **(C)** Axial post-contrast computed tomography (CT) image demonstrates that the smooth, homogeneous left apical mass has an attenuation value approximately equal to that of the subcutaneous adipose tissue (*arrow*).

◼ Differential Diagnosis

- ***Lipoma:*** The smooth, homogeneous character of the mass and its fat density are highly suggestive of a lipoma, a benign tumor.
- *Liposarcoma:* Rare lesions in pediatric patients, liposarcomas are often large (> 10 cm) and demonstrate thick septa and soft-tissue-density components, although neither CT nor magnetic resonance imaging (MRI) can definitively distinguish benign from malignant lesions.
- *Angiomyolipoma:* These fat-containing masses associated with tuberous sclerosis can arise outside the kidney in such locations as the liver, spleen, and lymph nodes, but they usually contain nonadipose tissue and are rarely found in children who do not have tuberous sclerosis.

◼ Essential Facts

- One or more lipomas are found in approximately 1% of the population.
- Lipomas are the most common soft-tissue tumors, and more than half are located in the subcutaneous tissues, where they demonstrate the so-called slippage sign because they are not attached to the subcutaneous fascia.
- Lipomas appear lucent on radiographic imaging.
- Lipomas demonstrate brightness equal to that of fat on CT and MRI.

◼ Other Imaging Findings

- Ultrasound can generally distinguish lipomas from cysts and more heterogeneous tumors.

✓ Pearls & ✗ Pitfalls

- ✓ Imaging is rarely indicated for subcutaneous lipoma.

Case 7

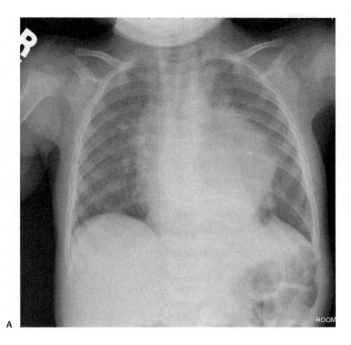

A

■ Clinical Presentation

A 3-year-old child with back pain and shortness of breath.

Further Work-up

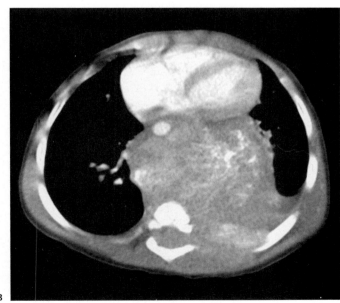

B

■ Imaging Findings

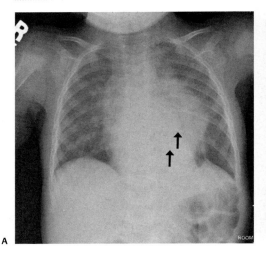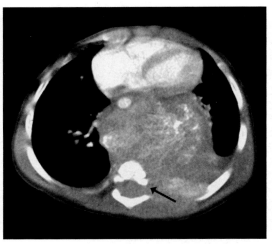

(A) Frontal chest radiograph demonstrates a large, predominately left-sided posterior mediastinal mass. The posterior location of the mass is apparent from several features: It obscures the margin of the descending aorta, and it is associated with increased distances between the posterior aspects of the lower ribs on the left in comparison with those on the right. Moreover, these ribs are eroded and narrowed medially (*arrows*). **(B)** Axial post-contrast computed tomography image demonstrates a large posterior mediastinal mass displacing the mediastinal structures anteriorly. It contains multiple calcifications and expands the left neural foramen as it invades the vertebral canal (*arrow*).

■ Differential Diagnosis

- **Neuroblastoma:** This is by far the most common posterior mediastinal malignancy in infants and children; the calcification and widening of the neural foramen are classic.
- *Other neural tumors:* These include ganglioneuroblastoma, ganglioneuroma, and neurofibroma, which are generally smaller and do not demonstrate such aggressive behavior.
- *Adenopathy:* Infection, such as tuberculosis, can produce a posterior mediastinal mass, although such masses generally do not grow so large or displace adjacent structures to this degree.

■ Essential Facts

- Neuroblastoma is the most common extracranial solid neoplasm and the most common abdominal malignancy in pediatric patients, as well as the third most common pediatric malignancy.
- The mean age at presentation is 2 years, with 40% of patients younger than 1 year and another 35% younger than 2 years.
- The prognosis·is best when the tumor is diagnosed in children younger than 1 year of age.
- Neuroblastoma arises from neural crest cells in the adrenal gland (40%), retroperitoneum (35%), and posterior mediastinum (20%).
- It tends to insinuate between adjacent structures, rather than simply displace them.
- The most common sites of metastasis are bone and liver.

■ Other Imaging Findings

- Bone scan: this is useful to detect cortical skeletal metastases.
- Meta-iodobenzylguanidine I 131 scan: Result is positive in approximately 75% of cases and helpful for assessing extent of disease before and after treatment; uptake is related to catecholamine production.
- Cranial imaging is important to detect central nervous system and skull involvement.

✓ Pearls & ✗ Pitfalls

- ✓ Skin metastases may appear as "blueberry muffin" lesions, and periorbital lesions may cause "raccoon eyes."
- ✓ Urine catecholamines will be elevated in 95% of patients.

Case 8

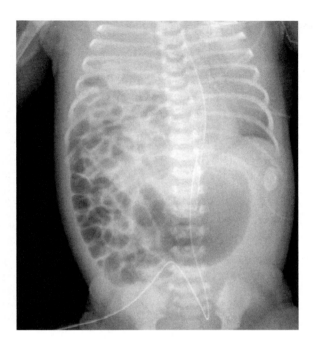

■ Clinical Presentation

A neonate with severe respiratory distress.

■ Imaging Findings

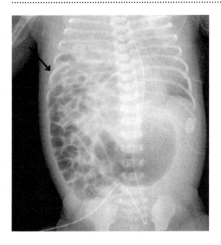

Frontal radiograph demonstrates cystic lucencies at the base of the right hemithorax, which appear continuous with abdominal bowel gas (*arrow*). The mediastinum is shifted to the left, and the gas-filled stomach is clearly located in the abdomen.

■ Differential Diagnosis

- **Congenital diaphragmatic hernia:** The bowel gas extending up from the abdomen, ipsilateral atelectasis, and contralateral mediastinal shift are all typical of congenital diaphragmatic hernia.
- *Congenital pulmonary adenomatoid malformation:* This may present as a multicystic mass in the base of the hemithorax but should not be continuous with bowel gas; the rate of change in appearance is considerably slower because the cysts do not represent bowel.
- *Cavitary pneumonia:* Although necrotizing pneumonia can produce multiple cavities in the lung base, this does not occur in the first few hours of life, when congenital diaphragmatic hernia typically presents.

■ Essential Facts

- Nearly 9 in 10 congenital diaphragmatic hernias are left-sided.
- They result from failure of the pleuroperitoneal folds to form and/or close in the second month of gestation.
- The presence of bowel in the thorax from this early stage results in pulmonary hypoplasia.
- Pulmonary hypertension is an important sequela of pulmonary hypoplasia and is often combined with hypoxemia and acidosis.
- Congenital diaphragmatic hernias are often detected at prenatal sonography.
- The incidence is approximately 1 in 2200 births.

✓ Pearls & ✗ Pitfalls

- ✓ Morgagni hernias, which are located anteromedially in the thorax and usually on the right, were described by Giovanni Battista Morgagni in 1761.
- ✓ Bochdalek hernias, which are located posterolaterally and account for approximately 90% of cases, were described by Victor Alexander Bochdalek in the mid-19th century.
- ✓ The lesion may be radiopaque initially because of the absence of gas in the bowel. If this persists with a right-sided lesion, it may indicate a hernia that contains only liver.
- ✓ There is a strong association with malrotation.
- ✓ Extracorporeal membrane oxygenation is often used to sustain the patient during the first week of life, when pulmonary hypertension tends to be the worst, before surgical repair.

Case 9

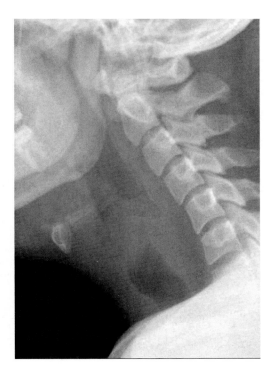

Clinical Presentation

A teenager with severe sore throat, fever, and drooling.

■ Imaging Findings

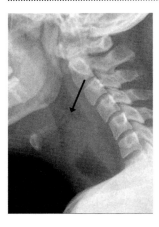

A lateral radiograph of the soft tissue of the neck demonstrates marked thickening of the epiglottis ("thumb sign," *arrow*) and aryepiglottic folds.

■ Differential Diagnosis

- **Epiglottitis:** The finding of marked thickening of the epiglottis and aryepiglottic folds is typical, particularly in a clinical setting that includes stridor, dysphagia, fever, and a toxic appearance.
- *Normal variant:* Sometimes called an *omega epiglottis*, this imaging artifact occurs when patients are positioned slightly obliquely so that both sides of the esophagus are seen adjacent to each other, but there is no thickening of the aryepiglottic folds.
- *Croup:* There may be narrowing of the subglottic airway ("steeple sign") on the frontal view, but the epiglottis and aryepiglottic folds themselves should be normal.

■ Essential Facts

- Epiglottitis usually has an infectious etiology, although other causes include thermal injury, trauma, chemical ingestion, and angioneurotic edema.
- Routine immunization against *Haemophilus influenzae* type b infection has raised the median age of patients, so that teenagers are affected more often than small children.
- The danger of acute airway occlusion makes this an emergent condition, requiring care by a medical professional skilled in airway management.

✓ Pearls & ✗ Pitfalls

- ✓ The threat of asphyxiation is generally related to swelling of the aryepiglottic folds, not the epiglottis itself.
- ✓ The age distribution is very different from that of croup, which usually occurs in the first 2 years of life.

Case 10

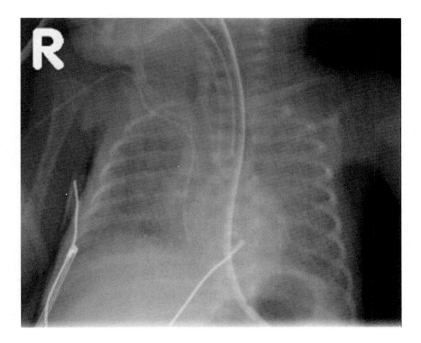

Clinical Presentation

An infant with persistent respiratory distress and poor breath sounds despite intubation.

■ Imaging Findings

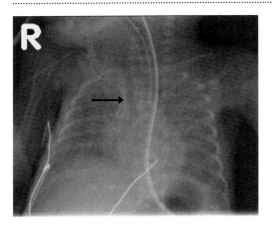

Frontal chest radiograph demonstrates underinflated lungs and the endotracheal tube paralleling the course of the esophageal tube, with the tracheal air column clearly positioned separately and to the right (*arrow*).

■ Differential Diagnosis

- **Esophageal intubation:** An endotracheal tube positioned in the esophagus can be very difficult to detect on frontal radiographs, but in this case seeing the endotracheal tube positioned lateral to the trachea establishes the diagnosis.
- *Bronchial intubation:* An endotracheal tube positioned too far caudally in one of the main bronchi (usually the right) can be associated with contralateral atelectasis and lack of breath sounds.
- *High position of the endotracheal tube:* An endotracheal tube positioned above the glottis can result in hypoventilation of the lungs, and in some cases the tip of the endotracheal tube may be above the top edge of the radiograph and thus not visualized.

■ Essential Facts

- Many esophageal intubations are detected clinically and corrected before radiography.
- Chest radiography is always indicated following endotracheal intubation to verify tube position.
- By the time the radiograph is seen by a radiologist, the problem has typically been corrected, but it is important to verify immediately that the physician, nurse, or respiratory therapist is aware of it.

✓ Pearls and ✗ Pitfalls

- ✓ Always evaluate the position of every line and tube on every radiograph.
- ✓ Look to make sure that the endotracheal tube follows the expected location of the trachea.
- ✓ Hypoinflated lungs and gaseous distention of the esophagus and stomach are typical findings in esophageal intubation.
- ✗ Do not fail to notify the clinical service immediately, as this condition can result in rapid deterioration.

Case 11

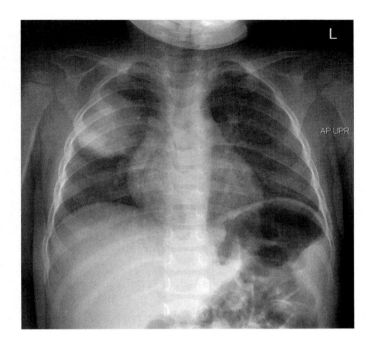

■ Clinical Presentation

A child with fever and cough.

■ Imaging Findings

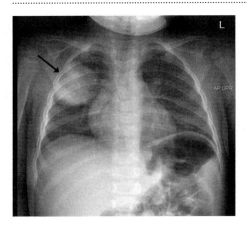

Frontal chest radiograph demonstrates a masslike opacity in the right upper lobe (*arrow*) with otherwise clear lungs.

■ Differential Diagnosis

- ***Round pneumonia:*** In the clinical setting of acute infection and because primary pulmonary malignancies are so rare in children, a round opacity in a child is most likely to represent a round pneumonia, a diagnosis supported in this case by the presence of air bronchograms in the medial portion of the lesion.
- *Bronchogenic cysts:* These lesions often appear as round masses, although they are typically located closer to the main airways and should not contain gas unless they have become infected.
- *Pulmonary metastasis:* Hematogenous metastases from lesions such as Wilms tumor and rhabdomyosarcoma often appear as round masses, although such lesions are typically multiple and do not contain air bronchograms.

■ Essential Facts

- As with community-acquired pneumonias in general, the most common agent is *Streptococcus pneumoniae.*
- In children between the ages of 1 month and 5 years, most community-acquired pneumonias are viral.
- Many bacterial pneumonias probably result from viral respiratory infection, which impairs the host defenses and is followed by bacterial superinfection.
- Chest radiography is the mainstay of diagnosis and is performed not only to look for pneumonia but also to rule out other processes (e.g., foreign body) and complications (e.g., large pleural effusions or empyema).

■ Other Imaging Findings

- In patients with typical clinical features of pneumonia, computed tomography is not indicated to rule out a neoplasm, although a follow-up chest radiograph may be obtained in 2 to 3 weeks to ensure resolution.

✓ Pearls & ✗ Pitfalls

- ✓ The greater frequency of round patterns of pneumonia in children is generally attributed to the immature state of conduits of collateral air drift in the lung (channels of Lambert and pores of Kohn).

Case 12

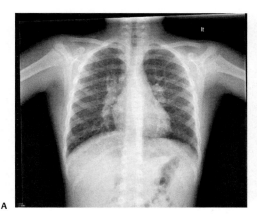

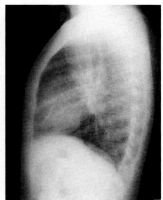

A

B

■ Clinical Presentation

A child with a history of cough and night sweats.

Further Work-up

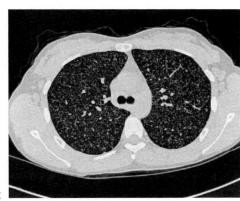

C

■ **Imaging Findings**

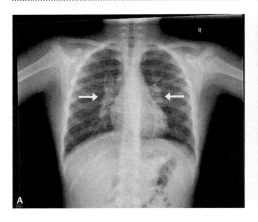 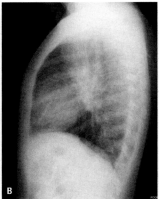 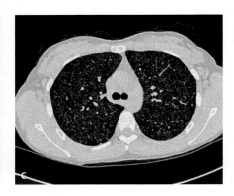

(A,B) Frontal and lateral chest radiographs demonstrate innumerable small pulmonary nodules bilaterally and hilar enlargement bilaterally (*arrows*), presumably reflecting adenopathy. **(C)** A high-resolution axial computed tomography image at the level of the tracheal bifurcation demonstrates innumerable pulmonary nodules bilaterally in a "miliary" pattern.

■ **Differential Diagnosis**

- **Tuberculosis:** The miliary pattern of pulmonary nodules with hilar adenopathy is highly suggestive of tuberculosis, particularly in the setting of cough and night sweats.
- *Other granulomatous disease:* In the appropriate geographic regions, histoplasmosis (midwestern United States) and coccidioidomycosis (southwestern United States) can exhibit a similar imaging pattern and clinical presentation.
- *Hypersensitivity pneumonitis:* This can manifest with centrilobular nodular opacities, caused by the inhalation of organic particulate matter including fungi, avian proteins, and dusts.

■ **Essential Facts**

- Tuberculosis is the most important infectious cause of death worldwide, infecting one-third of the human population.
- It is transmitted by respiratory droplets.
- Mycobacteria may lie dormant in granulomas and reactivate the infection many years later.
- Risk factors include exposure to an infected adult and contact with people from or travel to Asia, the Pacific Islands, Latin America, the Middle East, and Africa.
- Children in whom tuberculosis is suspected should undergo a tuberculin skin test.
- Chest radiographs should be obtained in all patients with a newly positive tuberculin skin test result; a positive chest radiograph establishes the diagnosis of tuberculosis.
- Treatment for tuberculosis typically involves at least three drugs, with a fourth drug added for multidrug-resistant disease.

✓ **Pearls & ✗ Pitfalls**

- ✓ Miliary tuberculosis is so named because of the resemblance of the tiny nodules to millet seeds.
- ✓ Other relatively common manifestations include meningitis, osteomyelitis, and arthritis.
- ✓ Patients remain infective for several weeks after commencing treatment.

Case 13

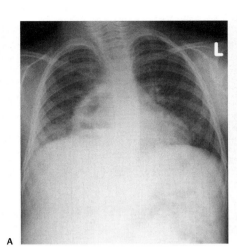
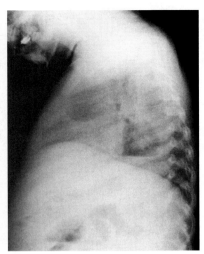

A   B

▣ Clinical Presentation
··

A child with chronic cough and recent fever.

■ Imaging Findings

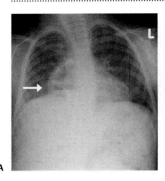 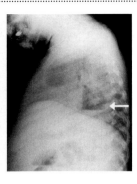

A   B

(A,B) Frontal and lateral chest radiographs demonstrate a large, thick-walled cystic mass in the right lower lobe containing a prominent air-fluid level (*arrows*).

■ Differential Diagnosis

• ***Congenital pulmonary adenomatous malformation (CPAM):*** This commonly presents as a mass lesion containing several large cysts or multiple small cysts, although it may rarely appear solid. In this case, the thickness of the wall and presence of fever suggest bacterial superinfection.
• *Necrotizing pneumonia:* A bacterial or fungal pneumonia may cavitate and appear as a thick-walled cyst with an air-fluid level, indistinguishable radiologically from an infected CPAM.
• *Hiatal hernia:* A large hiatal hernia can present as an air-fluid level containing a mass in the lower mediastinum, although this lesion appears to be centered in the right lower lobe.

■ Essential Facts

• A hamartoma consisting of abnormal terminal bronchiolar proliferation with a relative paucity of alveoli
• Bronchial communication present congenitally
• No lobar predilection
• Often detected on prenatal sonography
• At least three types:
  • Type 1: one or more large cysts measuring more than 2 cm in diameter
  • Type 2: numerous smaller macroscopic cysts
  • Type 3: appears solid on radiologic imaging
• Presentation arising from mass effect or infection (recurrent pneumonias in older children)

✓ Pearls & ✘ Pitfalls

✓ CPAM was formerly known as *congenital cystic adenomatous malformation.*
✓ There is a small long-term risk for malignant transformation. Because of this risk, combined with the risk for infection, many centers routinely resect asymptomatic lesions after the neonatal period.

Case 14

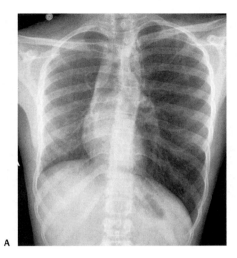

A

■ Clinical Presentation

An 18-year-old with cough and chest pain.

Further Work-up

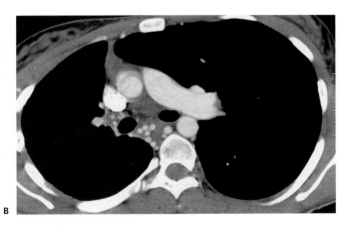

B

■ Imaging Findings

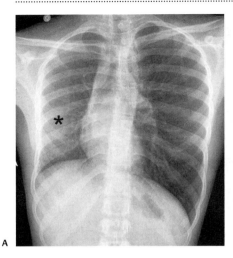

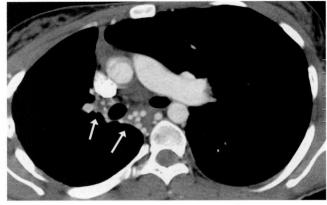

(A) On an anteroposterior view of the chest, the right lung is smaller than the left, and the heart and mediastinum are shifted to the right (*asterisk*). Additionally, the right hilar shadow is diminutive. **(B)** On an axial contrasted computed tomography (CT) image, the right hemithorax is smaller than the left, and the right pulmonary artery is not seen. Additionally, multiple small, enhancing vessels surround the right main bronchus (*arrows*).

■ Differential Diagnosis

- **Congenital absence of the right pulmonary artery:** The absent pulmonary artery is usually on the side opposite the aortic arch, and the ipsilateral lung is hypoplastic or absent. The small, enhancing vessels are collaterals that supply blood to the right lung.
- *Swyer-James syndrome:* In this syndrome, there is a hyperlucent and underperfused lung with a normal or decreased volume. The ipsilateral hilum is small but present. There is also air trapping on expiration, which is not seen in congenital absence of the right pulmonary artery.
- *Hypogenetic lung syndrome:* This is associated with right lung hypoplasia and anomalous pulmonary venous drainage. The pulmonary artery is usually present but small, although it can be absent or normal.

■ Essential Facts

- The patient is usually asymptomatic but can present with pulmonary hypertension in the contralateral lung, infection, exercise intolerance, hemoptysis, or congenital heart disease.
- Congenital absence of the right pulmonary artery usually occurs on the side opposite the aortic arch, and the ipsilateral lung is absent or hypoplastic.
- Absence of the left pulmonary artery is associated with a right arch without congenital heart disease. Absence of the right pulmonary artery is associated with a left arch and congenital heart disease (usually tetralogy of Fallot).

- A small, hyperlucent lung on the side opposite the aortic arch has an absent or small hilum and decreased pulmonary vascular markings. The mediastinum is shifted to the side of the absent artery.
- Ventilation-perfusion scanning demonstrates complete absence of perfusion to the affected lung with normal ventilation. There are no perfusion or ventilation defects in the contralateral lung.
- CT may demonstrate an aortopulmonary collateral network feeding the intrapulmonary vessels in the ipsilateral lung. The bronchial arteries, internal mammary arteries, and lateral thoracic artery may be enlarged.
- CT should demonstrate a normal bronchial branching pattern and may show bronchiectasis as a result of recurrent infections.

✓ Pearls & ✗ Pitfalls

✗ Congenital absence of the right pulmonary artery is easily confused with Swyer-James syndrome; however, there should be no air trapping, as is seen in Swyer-James syndrome.

Case 15

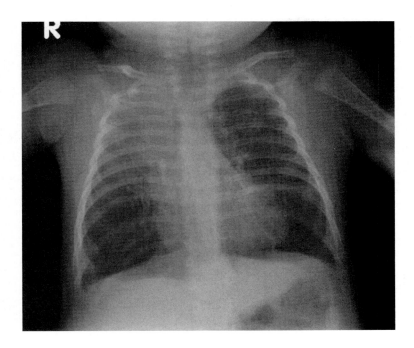

Clinical Presentation

An infant with wheezing and respiratory distress.

■ Imaging Findings

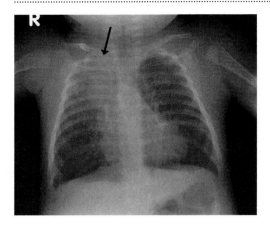

Frontal chest radiograph demonstrates hyperinflation with patchy air space opacities bilaterally, most prominent in the right upper lobe (*arrow*).

■ Differential Diagnosis

- **Viral bronchiolitis:** Classic findings include hyperinflation, areas of atelectasis and hyperinflation, and predominately perihilar air space and interstitial opacities.
- *Pneumonia:* Viral bronchiolitis and pneumonia exist along a continuum, but bacterial pneumonias typically demonstrate more focal air space disease and are more likely to be accompanied by pleural effusion.
- *Asthma:* In infants and small children, viral bronchiolitis and asthma are radiographically indistinguishable.

■ Essential Facts

- The most common causes are rhinovirus, respiratory syncytial virus, and parainfluenza virus.
- Infection results in airway inflammation, increased mucous production, and the formation of intraluminal cellular debris, resulting in airway occlusion.
- Airway narrowing is a more serious problem in smaller children because tiny decreases in luminal diameter produce disproportionately large reductions in cross-sectional area.
- Seasonal increases in incidence are noted, with a peak in winter.

✓ Pearls & ✗ Pitfalls

- ✓ Chest radiography is most important to rule out other causes of the presentation, such as bacterial pneumonia and airway foreign body.
- ✓ Once the diagnosis is established, radiography is used to assess support apparatus and rule out complications such as pneumothorax.

Case 16

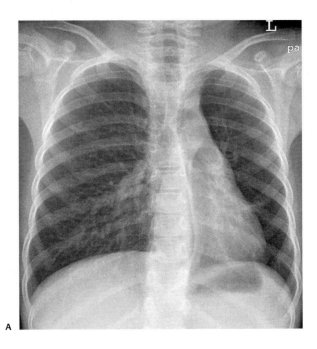

A

Clinical Presentation

A 10-year-old boy with cough.

Further Work-up

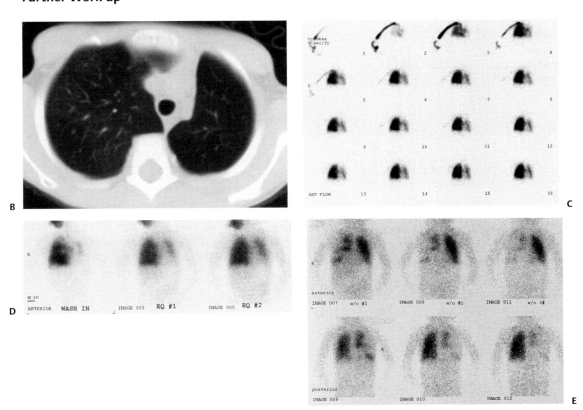

Imaging Findings

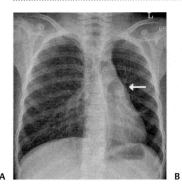
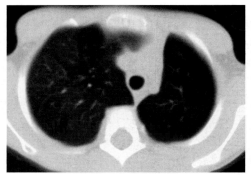
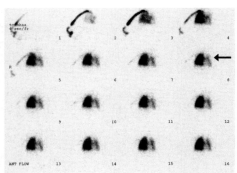
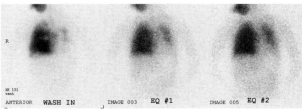
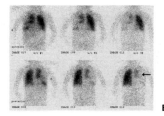

(A) Frontal chest radiograph demonstrates a small, hyperlucent left lung with diminished pulmonary vascularity. Left hilar vessels are present (*arrow*). **(B)** Axial computed tomography (CT) image confirms small left lung with decreased vascularity. **(C)** A nuclear medicine perfusion scan demonstrates markedly diminished perfusion of the left lung (*arrow*). **(D,E)** Nuclear medicine ventilation scans demonstrate decreased aeration of the left lung with air trapping (*arrow*).

Differential Diagnosis

- **Swyer-James syndrome:** A small, hyperlucent lung that has a small hilum and exhibits decreased perfusion and ventilation with air trapping is consistent with Swyer-James syndrome.
- *Pulmonary artery hypoplasia/agenesis:* In this disease, the ventilation washout images would be normal.
- *Congenital lobar emphysema (CLE):* In CLE, the larger lung is hyperlucent, and there would be abnormal ventilation in the larger lung.

Essential Facts

- Swyer-James syndrome is likely due to adenoviral or other infection causing bronchiolitis obliterans before the age of 8 years, when the full complement of alveoli has formed. This leads to obliteration of the distal bronchioles, fewer alveoli, and hypoplasia of the vasculature.
- It can lead to chronic lung disease.
- Lung hyperlucency, underperfusion, and air trapping with a normal to decreased lung volume are characteristic. The ipsilateral hilum is small but present.
- Imaging findings appear a few months to a few years after the inciting infection.
- Serial radiographs show little growth in the affected lung.

- CT: Expiratory imaging should be obtained to demonstrate air trapping.
- Treatment involves maximizing the function of the normal lung with such measures as avoiding smoking and inhalational injury.

Other Imaging Findings

- Fluoroscopy: During rapid expiration, the mediastinum swings sharply toward the normal lung and the hemidiaphragm rises sharply on the normal side. The hemidiaphragm on the abnormal side will have much less movement because of air trapping.

✓ Pearls & ✗ Pitfalls

- ✓ Hyperlucency is caused by decreased perfusion rather than increased ventilation.
- ✗ When Swyer-James syndrome involves just a lobe, it may be mistaken for congenital lobar emphysema.

Case 17

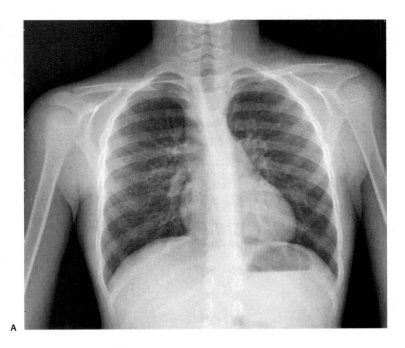

A

Clinical Presentation

A child with episodic shortness of breath.

Further Work-up

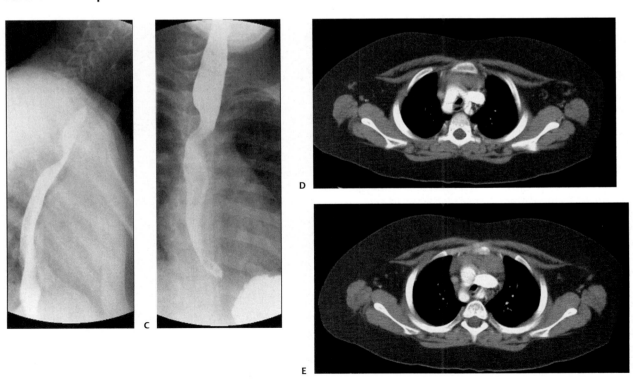

B

C

D

E

■ Imaging Findings

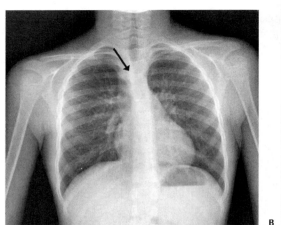
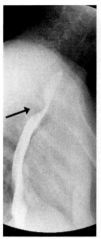
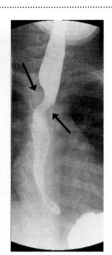
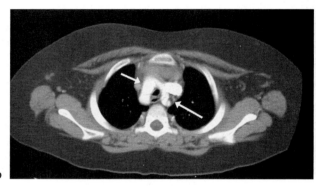
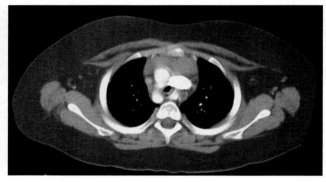

(A) Frontal chest radiograph demonstrates clear lungs and a normal cardiac silhouette. However, there is a right-sided impression on the tracheal air column at the level of the aortic arch (*arrow*). **(B,C)** Lateral image from a barium esophagogram demonstrates a prominent, smooth posterior impression on the upper esophagus (*arrow*), whereas the frontal view shows bilateral impressions, the one on the right located cranial to the one on the left (*arrows*). **(D,E)** Post-contrast axial computed tomography images of the chest demonstrate right- and left-sided aortas (*arrows*), which impinge on the anterior aspect of the trachea and posterior aspect of the esophagus, a so-called vascular ring.

■ Differential Diagnosis

- **Double aortic arch:** The finding of right and left aortic arches connected to both the ascending and descending aorta is diagnostic.
- *Right aortic arch with aberrant left subclavian artery:* May appear identical on plain radiographs and esophagography but shows no left aortic arch on cross-sectional imaging.
- *Esophageal duplication:* May impinge on the trachea and esophagus on radiography and barium studies but does not enhance with intravenous administration of contrast.

■ Essential Facts

- Persistence of both embryonic aortic arches
- Most common symptomatic vascular ring
- Each arch with its own carotid and subclavian arteries
- Right arch crossing behind esophagus to join left-sided arch, descending aorta
- Increased incidence of congenital heart disease

✓ Pearls & ✗ Pitfalls

- ✓ The condition often presents with stridor.
- ✓ Cross-sectional images above the arch show four arteries instead of the usual three.

Case 18

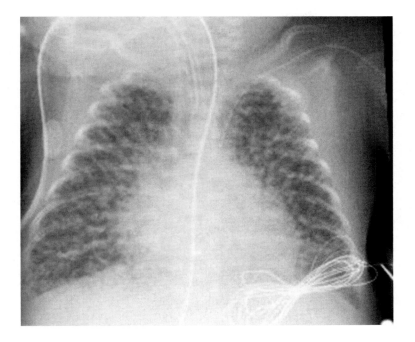

■ **Clinical Presentation**

A premature newborn on a ventilator.

■ Imaging Findings

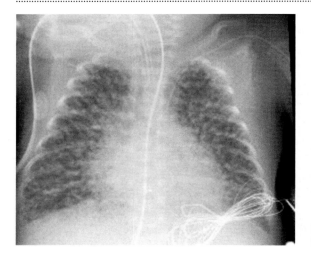

Frontal chest radiograph demonstrates extensive linear and bubble-like lucencies throughout both lungs that radiate from the hila to the periphery.

■ Differential Diagnosis

- *Pulmonary interstitial emphysema (PIE):* Bubble-like or linear lucencies that radiate from the hila in a premature infant on a ventilator are consistent with PIE.
- *Partially treated surfactant deficiency disease (SDD):* This can be difficult to differentiate from PIE. When SDD is treated with surfactant, there may be re-expansion of some alveoli, but not others, in a pattern that mimics PIE. It is helpful to know when surfactant was administered.
- *Developing bronchopulmonary dysplasia (BPD):* This can appear similar to PIE but is usually of gradual onset, whereas PIE is more abrupt. Additionally, PIE typically occurs within the first week of life, and BPD findings appear later.

■ Essential Facts

- Abnormal collections of air in the peribronchial and perivascular spaces are secondary to increased alveolar pressure and rupture (barotrauma).
- Air may further dissect through the interstitium, causing pneumomediastinum or pneumothorax.
- PIE occurs in ventilated infants, usually during the first several days of life but almost always during the first week of life.
- It may be asymptomatic but can cause difficulty in ventilation.
- It is often treated by adjusting the ventilator settings or switching from conventional ventilation to high-frequency ventilation.
- Plain films: Lucencies may be focal or diffuse. On consecutive radiographs, the lucencies are typically transient. The lucencies and volume of the involved lung may not change with respiration.

■ Other Imaging Findings

- Computed tomography: Not needed to evaluate typical PIE; however, it can be obtained to differentiate PIE from other lucent lung lesions. In PIE, air engulfs the pulmonary vessels, which appear as a round soft-tissue density surrounded by abnormal lucency.

✓ Pearls & ✗ Pitfalls

- ✓ PIE can be the first sign of impending complications of air block, including pneumothorax and pneumomediastinum.
- ✗ If PIE affects just one lobe, or if it persists and forms an air-filled mass, it can appear similar to congenital cystic adenomatoid malformation or congenital lobar emphysema.

Case 19

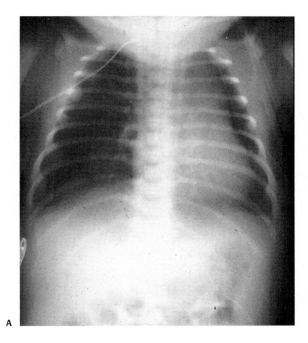

■ Clinical Presentation

An infant with repeated bouts of respiratory difficulty.

Further Work-up

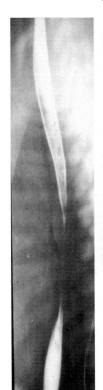

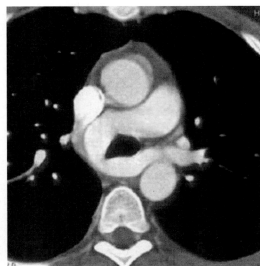

◼ Imaging Findings

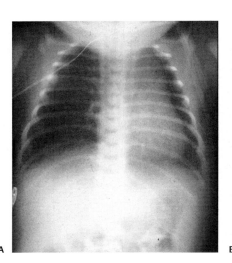
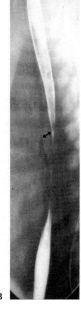
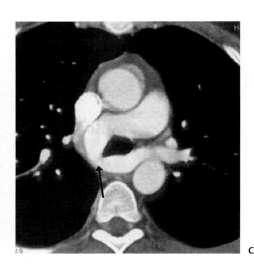

A   B   C

(A) A frontal chest radiograph demonstrates leftward shift of the mediastinum, suggesting hyperinflation of the right lung.
(B) A lateral barium esophagogram reveals a focal mass effect on the posterior aspect of the trachea and the anterior aspect of the esophagus (*arrow*). **(C)** Axial post-contrast computed tomography (CT) scan of the chest at the level of right pulmonary artery reveals an anomalous origin of the left pulmonary artery, which is arising from the right pulmonary artery (*arrow*) and then coursing leftward between the trachea and esophagus.

◼ Differential Diagnosis

- ***Pulmonary sling:*** This is the only relatively common vascular anomaly that lies between the trachea and esophagus, thus creating an impression on the anterior aspect of the esophagus. The CT appearance is pathognomonic.
- *Foregut malformation:* Other nonvascular congenital malformations, such as bronchogenic cyst and esophageal duplication cyst, can present as a mass between the trachea and esophagus, although neither would exhibit vascular enhancement.
- *Lymphadenopathy:* Enlarged lymph nodes could present as a mediastinal mass in this location.

◼ Essential Facts

- Pulmonary sling typically presents with respiratory symptoms such as stridor.
- It is associated with other anomalies, such as tracheomalacia, complete tracheal rings, and congenital heart disease.
- In some cases, the anomalous pulmonary artery may supply only a portion of the left lung.

✓ Pearls & ✗ Pitfalls

- ✓ This is the only vascular anomaly associated with asymmetric pulmonary inflation.
- ✓ On diagnosis, echocardiography is indicated to rule out associated congenital heart disease.

Case 20

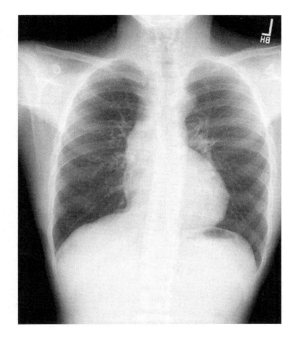

■ Clinical Presentation

A hypertensive teenager with lower blood pressures in the lower extremities than in the upper extremities.

■ **Imaging Findings**

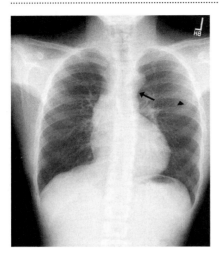

Frontal chest radiograph demonstrates ectasia of the ascending aorta and an enlarged aortic knob with a "notch" between the aortic knob and the proximal descending thoracic aorta (*arrow*). There is also mild rib notching, best seen in the posterior aspect of the left sixth rib (*arrowhead*).

■ **Differential Diagnosis**

- ***Coarctation of the aorta:*** The findings of a prominent ascending aorta, enlarged aortic knob, notch between the aortic knob and proximal descending thoracic aorta, and rib notching are highly suggestive of coarctation of the aorta.
- *Aortic stenosis:* This lesion is associated with post-stenotic dilatation of the ascending aorta, but isolated aortic stenosis should not demonstrate the other clinical and radiographic findings seen in this case.
- *Pseudocoarctation:* A condition associated with elongation and "kinking" of the aorta, pseudocoarctation causes a radiographically prominent aortic knob but no true stenosis or blood pressure gradient.

■ **Essential Facts**

- Most cases are located adjacent to the ductus arteriosus/ligamentum arteriosum (juxtaductal).
- Coarctation of the aorta is likely associated with the contraction of smooth muscle at the time of closure of the ductus arteriosus.
- This condition accounts for 6 to 8% of all congenital cardiac defects.
- It is three times more common in males.
- It is associated with bicuspid aortic valve (with increased probability of the development of aortic stenosis) in 50% of cases.
- Coarctation is also associated with ventricular septal defect, patent ductus arteriosus, and mitral stenosis.
- An increased incidence of cerebral aneurysms is noted in these patients.
- Rib notching is caused by the development of intercostal collaterals.

■ **Other Imaging Findings**

- Computed tomography is excellent for detection but provides little hemodynamic assessment.
- Magnetic resonance imaging permits a more accurate assessment of the hemodynamic effects, such as pressure gradients, and is useful for postoperative follow-up.
- Echocardiography is good for hemodynamic assessment.
- Angiography is increasingly reserved for intervention (balloon angioplasty).

✓ **Pearls & ✗ Pitfalls**

- ✓ Rib notching may be the only radiographic finding in clinically unsuspected cases.
- ✓ Decreased renal perfusion may exacerbate hypertension through the renin-angiotensin system.

Case 21

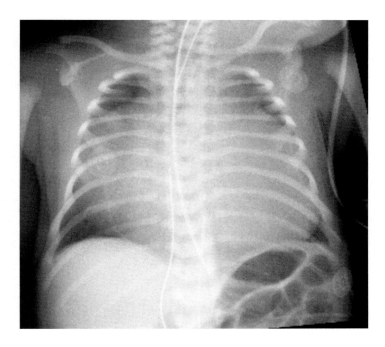

■ Clinical Presentation

Severe cyanosis in a newborn.

■ Imaging Findings

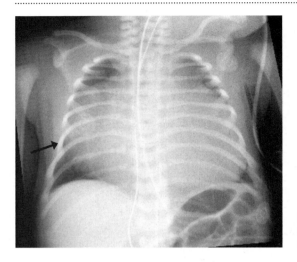

Frontal chest radiograph demonstrates massive "boxlike" cardiomegaly with marked convexity of the right border of the heart (*arrow*). Pulmonary vascularity appears to be diminished.

■ Differential Diagnosis

- *Ebstein anomaly (EA):* Massive cardiomegaly with marked convexity of the right border of the heart, as well as diminished pulmonary vascularity, is typical of EA.
- *Pulmonary atresia with intact ventricular septum:* This lesion can have an identical appearance, with massive right atriomegaly arising from tricuspid insufficiency.
- *Pericardial effusion:* Large pericardial effusions can mimic severe cardiomegaly, although they should not be associated with cyanosis or diminished pulmonary vascularity.

■ Essential Facts

- Displacement of the tricuspid valve into the right ventricle, with "atrialization" of the ventricle and tricuspid insufficiency, causes right atriomegaly and volume overload of the right side of the heart.
- EA is associated with maternal lithium use.
- EA is associated with numerous other cardiac problems, such as atrial septal defect and reentrant dysrhythmias.
- The severity varies widely, with some patients not presenting until adolescence or adulthood.

■ Other Imaging Findings

- Echocardiography is diagnostic.
- Magnetic resonance imaging is useful in evaluating chamber volumes and ejection fractions.

✓ Pearls and ✗ Pitfalls

- ✓ Infants with Ebstein anomaly generally present with cyanosis and/or heart failure.
- ✗ A large pericardial effusion can mimic Ebstein anomaly.

Case 22

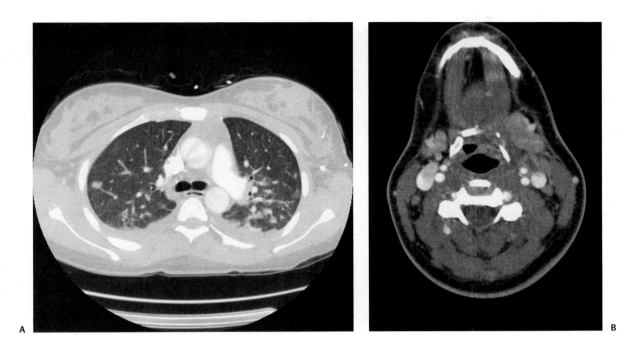

A   B

■ Clinical Presentation

A child with severe sore throat, fever, swollen neck, and respiratory distress.

Imaging Findings

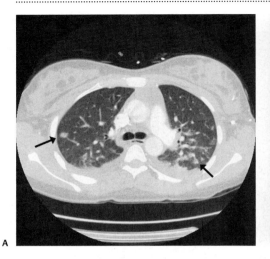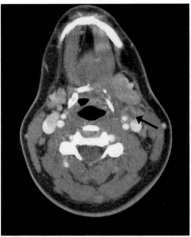

A   B

(A) Axial lung window computed tomography (CT) image of the chest demonstrates bilateral nodular air space opacities (*arrows*) and pleural effusions. On subsequent imaging, cavitation was noted in some of the nodular air space opacities. (B) Axial post-contrast CT image of the neck demonstrates inflammation and early abscess formation in the left lateral pharyngeal tissues and a filling defect in a branch of the left internal jugular vein (*arrow*).

Differential Diagnosis

- *Lemierre syndrome:* This disorder is defined as infection of the lateral pharyngeal space and septic thrombosis of the jugular vein, which may be complicated by septic pulmonary emboli.
- *Wegener granulomatosis:* This is a necrotizing vasculitis that can cause cavitary pulmonary nodules and is also associated with necrotizing granulomas in the upper respiratory tract and focal glomerulonephritis.
- *Laryngotracheal papillomatosis:* This condition also may present with cavitary lung nodules but is not associated with pharyngitis, thrombophlebitis, or pleural effusions.

Essential Facts

- Lemierre syndrome is most common in children and young adults, who may present with high fever, respiratory distress, and septic shock.
- Suppurative infection spreads from the lateral pharyngeal space into the carotid sheath, causing thrombophlebitis of the jugular vein.
- It is most often associated with *Fusobacterium necrophorum*, an anaerobe normally present in the oral cavity.

Other Imaging Findings

- Chest radiograph demonstrates typical findings of septic emboli.
- Neck sonography shows jugular thrombosis and adjacent inflammation.
- CT is generally best for the assessment of neck and chest disease.

✓ Pearls and ✗ Pitfalls

- ✓ When chest imaging demonstrates possible septic emboli, consider possible sites of phlebitis as well as endocarditis.
- ✗ Remember that pulmonary nodules in children are much less likely to reflect malignancy than in adults.

Case 23

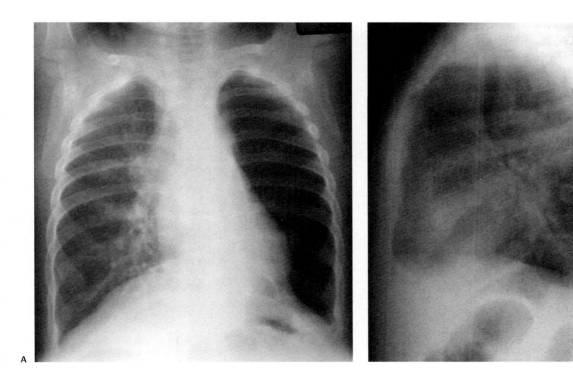

A

B

■ Clinical Presentation

An 8-year-old boy with chest pain and difficulty swallowing.

Further Work-up

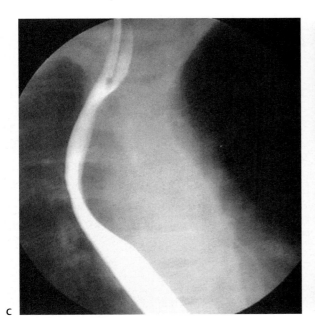

C

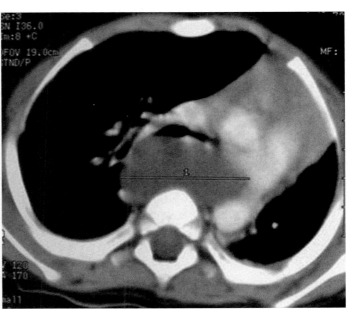

D

■ Imaging Findings

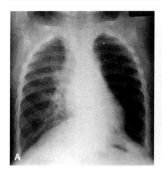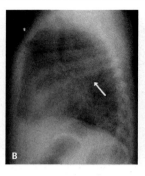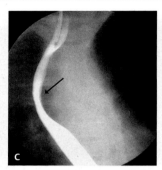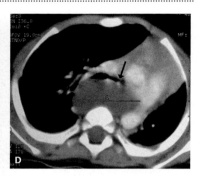

(A,B) Frontal chest radiograph demonstrates right paratracheal opacity. The left lung is hyperlucent. Lateral chest radiograph demonstrates a large mass posterior to the trachea (*arrow*), associated with tracheal narrowing. **(C)** Esophagogram demonstrates that the esophagus is displaced to the right by an extramural mass (*arrow*). **(D)** Axial post-contrast computed tomography (CT) image shows a large, low-density mass at the level of the carina. It narrows the left main bronchus (*arrow*). The right lung is now hyper-expanded.

■ Differential Diagnosis

- **Bronchogenic cyst:** All of the preceding findings are typical of a bronchogenic cyst.
- *Esophageal duplication/neurenteric cyst:* This can be difficult to differentiate from a bronchogenic cyst, although bronchogenic cysts are typically middle mediastinal in location and esophageal cysts are typically posterior mediastinal. On an esophagogram, esophageal cysts are typically intramural.
- *Necrotic lymphadenopathy:* Lymphadenopathy is usually multilobular, not typically with fluid density, and would show some contrast enhancement.

■ Essential Facts

- Bronchogenic cysts result from abnormal ventral budding of the tracheobronchial tree very early in gestation.
- Infants may present with respiratory distress. Older children may have chest pain or dysphagia. The lesions may also be found incidentally.
- Bronchogenic cysts may become infected.
- Surgical resection is recommended.
- The lesion is typically a well-defined, round/oval paratracheal or subcarinal cystic mass. Approximately 15% of them are found within the lung parenchyma.
- They can be detected on prenatal ultrasound.
- Plain radiographs: These show a well-defined, soft-tissue-density mass with smooth borders.
- CT: The lesion can be aqueous to proteinaceous in density. The thin wall should be nonenhancing or minimally enhancing. If the cyst is infected, the wall will be thicker and enhance.

■ Other Imaging Findings

- T2 and short inversion recovery magnetic resonance images show high signal intensity, almost always equal to or greater than that of cerebrospinal fluid.

✓ Pearls & ✗ Pitfalls

- ✓ Neurenteric cysts are associated with vertebral anomalies.
- ✓ Esophageal duplication cysts are typically intramural lesions.
- ✗ A bronchogenic cyst can be difficult to distinguish from an esophageal duplication/neurenteric cyst.

Case 24

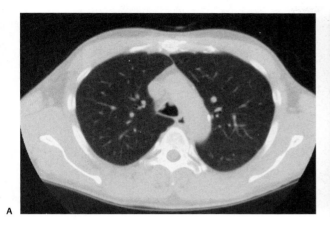 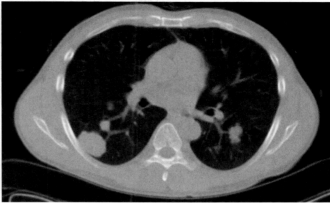

A   B

■ Clinical Presentation

A 4-year-old with hoarseness.

■ Imaging Findings

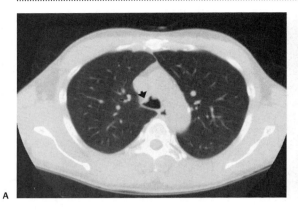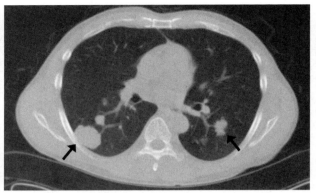

A   B

(A,B) Axial computed tomography (CT) images demonstrate multiple soft-tissue masses throughout both lungs (*arrows*). Notice the mural soft-tissue mass in the trachea (*arrowhead*).

■ Differential Diagnosis

- ***Papillomatosis:*** Soft-tissue masses within the airway as well as nodules in the lungs indicate papillomatosis.
- *Metastatic disease:* Wilms tumor frequently metastasizes to the lung, but the airway is not usually involved.
- *Invasive fungal disease:* These soft-tissue masses may have a ground-glass halo and occur in immunocompromised individuals. Also, they do not involve the trachea.

■ Essential Facts

- Perinatal transmission of the human papillomavirus from mother to child leads to benign tumors of the respiratory system and less commonly the digestive system.
- The mean age at diagnosis is 4 years.
- The most common signs/symptoms are voice changes, weak cry, wheezing/stridor, and complete airway obstruction.
- Frequent recurrences/exacerbations are common.
- Lung lesions usually grow over decades. Approximately 2% degenerate to squamous cell carcinoma.
- Repeated debulking by laser ablation of airway/laryngeal lesions is common.
- Interferon and antiviral agents may slow growth but are not curative.
- Tracheostomy may be needed.
- CT: Lesions are distributed predominantly in the posterior aspect of the lower lobes and are associated with bronchiectasis, atelectasis, and secondary infection. Malignant degeneration is suggested by a large mass with heterogeneous enhancement and lymphadenopathy.
- Soft-tissue growths in the larynx and tracheobronchial tree are associated with multiple round lung nodules that may show cavitation.

■ Other Imaging Findings

- Plain film: nodularity can often be seen in the trachea and bronchi.
- Fluoroscopy: this may be used to determine if soft-tissue masses in the trachea are due to secretions.

✓ Pearls & ✗ Pitfalls

- ✓ Papillomatosis is the most common cause of laryngeal tumors in children. Fewer than 1% spread to involve the lungs.
- ✓ Air-fluid levels within the lung cavities suggest superinfection.
- ✗ Manipulation of the lesions increases the risk for dissemination.

Case 25

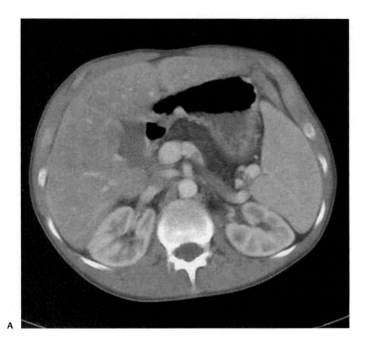

A

■ Clinical Presentation

A 17-year-old girl with frequent respiratory infections.

Further Work-up

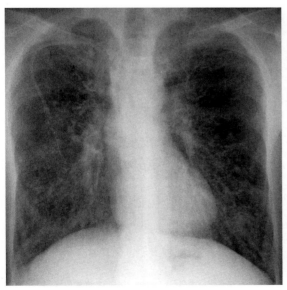

B

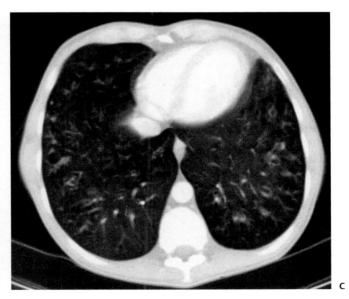

C

◼ Imaging Findings

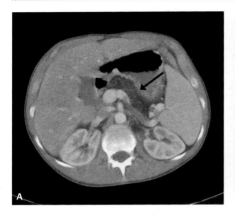 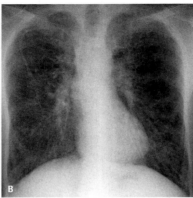 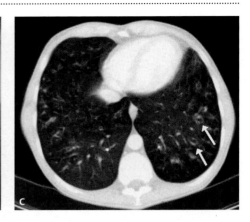

(A) Axial post-contrast computed tomography (CT) image of the abdomen demonstrates fatty replacement of the pancreas (*arrow*). **(B)** Frontal chest radiograph demonstrates bronchiectasis with hyperinflation of the lungs. A chest port is present. **(C)** Lung window CT image confirms the bronchiectasis (*arrows*).

◼ Differential Diagnosis

- **Cystic fibrosis (CF):** The combination of fatty replacement of the pancreas and bronchiectasis makes the diagnosis.
- *Schwachman-Diamond syndrome:* Although this disease can manifest as lipomatosis of the pancreas, bronchiectasis is not seen. Abnormal bony findings and short stature are typical.
- *Steroid therapy/Cushing syndrome:* This can cause pancreatic lipomatosis, but not bronchiectasis.

◼ Essential Facts

- This autosomal-recessive disease causes dysfunction of the exocrine glands, leading to thick mucus and reduced mucociliary transport.
- CF affects the lungs (recurrent infections), intestinal tract (meconium ileus, malabsorption), hepatobiliary system (cirrhosis, varices), pancreas (steatorrhea), and urogenital system (delayed sexual development).
- CF can present at any time from gestation to young adulthood.
- The prevalence is highest in Caucasians.
- The diagnosis is made by the sweat chloride test.
- Treatment consists of pancreatic enzymes, respiratory therapies.
- Prognosis: Fatal pulmonary complications develop in nearly all patients, but survival into the 3rd and 4th decades is increasingly common.
- Imaging findings in the lungs reflect extensive airway (rather than air space) involvement and include bronchiectasis (worst in upper lobes), mucous plugging, hyperinflation, atelectasis, and later spontaneous pneumothorax and pneumonia.

- The hila may be enlarged as the consequence of lymphadenopathy or dilatation of the pulmonary arteries.
- Imaging findings in the gastrointestinal tract include meconium ileus, meconium plug syndrome, intussusception, thick duodenal folds, fatty infiltration of the liver, biliary cirrhosis, atrophy, and fatty replacement of the pancreas.
- Other findings include wasting of the soft tissues, radiolucent metaphyseal bands, and opaque paranasal sinuses.

✓ Pearls & ✗ Pitfalls

- ✓ Infants with CF often present with meconium ileus.
- ✗ On CT, it is easy to miss what is not there. Always look for each organ on at least one axial image.

Case 26

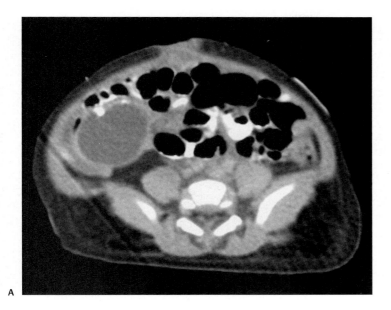

A

■ Clinical Presentation

A child with a palpable abdominal mass.

Further Work-up

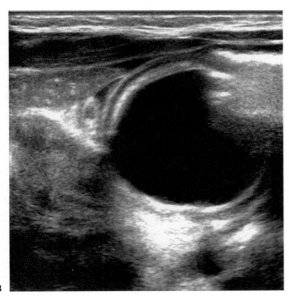

B

■ Imaging Findings

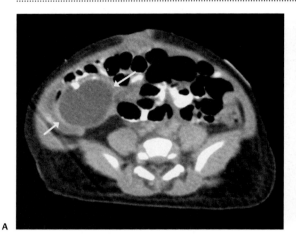 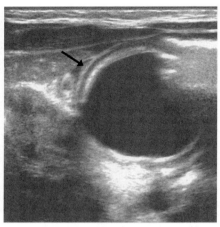

A   B

(A) Axial computed tomography image of the abdomen after oral and intravenous administration of contrast demonstrates a cystic lesion in the right side of the abdomen adjacent to bowel (*arrows*). The wall of the lesion demonstrates mild contrast enhancement, but the lumen does not fill with oral contrast material. **(B)** Transverse sonogram of the right side of the abdomen demonstrates a cystic lesion with a well-defined wall that exhibits an echogenic inner layer, a hypoechoic middle layer, and an echogenic outer layer (*arrow*).

■ Differential Diagnosis

- **Duplication cyst:** The finding of an echogenic mucosa, hypoechoic muscularis propria, and echogenic serosa ("gastrointestinal signature") in the wall of a cystic lesion is diagnostic for a duplication cyst of the gastrointestinal tract.
- *Mesenteric cyst:* These cysts are also found adjacent to bowel, but their walls do not exhibit the gastrointestinal signature pattern of echogenicity.
- *Lymphatic malformation:* Often has multiple septa and lacks the gastrointestinal signature.

■ Essential Facts

- Duplication cysts are congenital lesions that usually present in the first 2 years of life with pain, mass, or obstruction.
- They can arise from any part of the alimentary canal, with 75% located in the abdomen and 25% in the thorax.
- Many contain gastric mucosa. Acid secretion can result in mucosal inflammation, ulceration, hemorrhage, and perforation.
- Lesions without gastric or pancreatic tissue may secrete mucus, which accounts for their increase in size over time.
- They may also present by compressing adjacent structures or acting as a lead point for intussusception.

✓ Pearls & ✗ Pitfalls

- ✓ If the cyst is associated with a vertebral and/or spinal anomaly, think of neurenteric cyst.
- ✓ The cyst contents need not be anechoic and may contain debris.
- ✓ Some duplication cysts may communicate with adjacent bowel.

Case 27

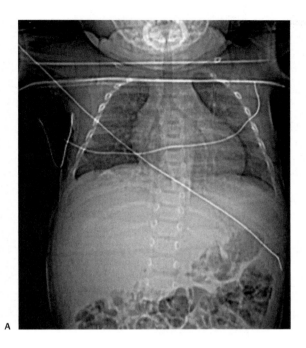

A

■ Clinical Presentation

A newborn with an abdominal mass.

Further Work-up

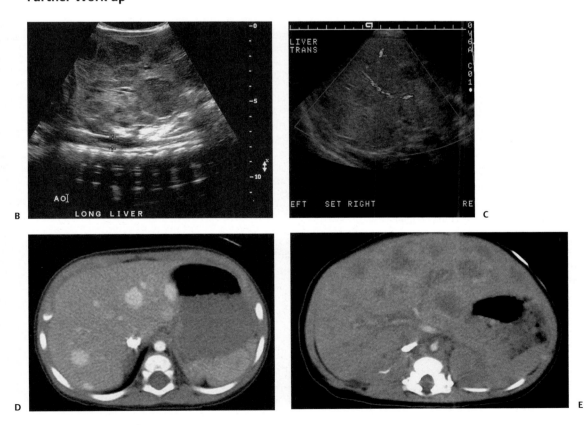

■ Imaging Findings

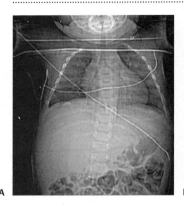
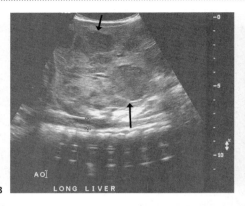
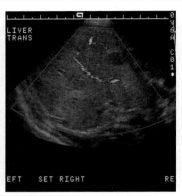

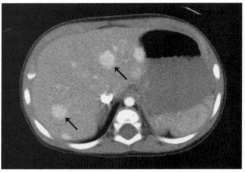
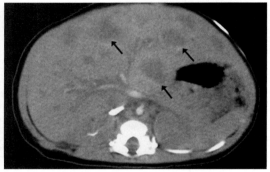

(A) Frontal radiograph of the chest demonstrates cardiomegaly and hepatomegaly. **(B,C)** Gray-scale and Doppler images of the liver demonstrate multiple hypoechoic lesions (*arrows*). There is high flow around and within the lesion. **(D,E)** Early and late post-contrast axial computed tomography (CT) images demonstrate a difference in the caliber of the aorta above and below the celiac artery, as well as multiple hypodense, intensely enhancing lesions in the liver (*arrows*).

■ Differential Diagnosis

- ***Hemangioendotheliomatosis:*** These findings are characteristic of hemangioendotheliomatosis.
- *Metastatic disease:* Metastatic neuroblastoma could have this appearance, but the caliber of the aorta should not change, and no primary lesion is identified.
- *Hepatoblastoma:* This tends to be a well-defined, solitary mass that can be hypervascular.

■ Essential Facts

- A benign, endothelium-lined vascular mass in the liver may cause arteriovenous shunting or consumptive coagulopathy.
- In 75% of cases, the presentation is before 6 months of age. The female-to-male ratio is 2:1.
- Signs and symptoms include hepatomegaly, high-output congestive heart failure, and consumptive coagulopathy (Kasabach-Merritt syndrome).
- Many patients also have cutaneous hemangiomas.
- The lesions usually involute spontaneously over months to years.
- Severely symptomatic lesions are treated with high-dose steroids, interferon alpha, embolization, or resection.
- Masses may be solitary, multiple, or diffusely infiltrative.

- Plain film: May have fine calcifications.
- Ultrasound: Nonspecific, variable appearance; usually discrete masses; caliber of aorta may abruptly decrease below level of the celiac axis.
- CT: Usually low attenuation before contrast but may have central high density due to hemorrhage or calcification; tend to enhance like adult hemangiomas; however, central enhancement can be absent in larger lesions, and smaller lesions may enhance completely.

■ Other Imaging Findings

- Magnetic resonance imaging: T1—low signal compared with normal liver, may have blood products; T2—high signal, may have flow voids and feeding vessels.
- Angiography: vascular mass with arteriovenous shunting and abnormal pooling, dilated hepatic artery and veins.

✓ Pearls & ✗ Pitfalls

- ✓ Consider hemangioendothelioma in an infant with congestive heart failure and a large liver on a plain film.
- ✓ Look for the change in the caliber of the aorta.
- ✗ Appearances can vary (single, multiple, or infiltrative; calcified or noncalcified), as can patterns of enhancement.

Case 28

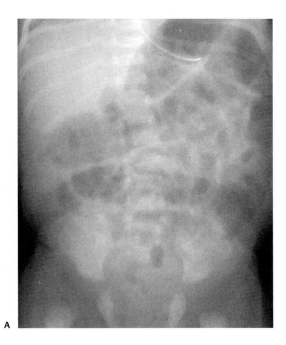

A

■ Clinical Presentation

A neonate with failure to pass meconium.

Further Work-up

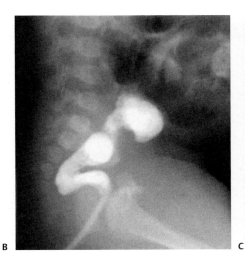

B

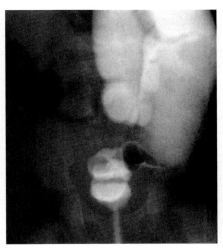

C

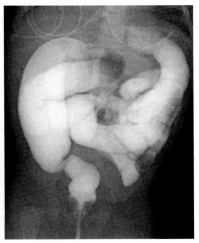

D

■ Imaging Findings

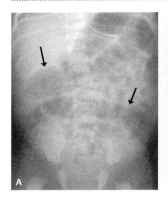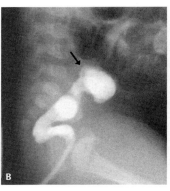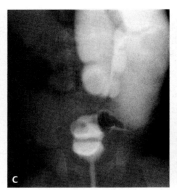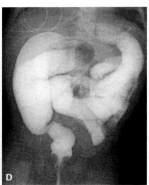

(A) Abdominal radiograph demonstrates mildly gaseous, distended bowel loops throughout the abdomen (*arrows*) with a nondistended rectum. **(B–D)** Contrast enema shows a narrow, poorly distensible rectum with a transition zone (*arrow*).

■ Differential Diagnosis

- **Hirschsprung disease:** These findings are typical of Hirschsprung disease.
- *Meconium plug:* Rectosigmoid ratio should be greater than 1; small-caliber left colon; usually has multiple colonic filling defects (meconium); may pass plugs during enema.
- *Meconium ileus:* Rectosigmoid ratio should be greater than 1, and there should be a microcolon with a meconium-filled terminal ileum.

■ Essential Facts

- Failure of migration of neural crest cells early in gestation leads to absence of the myenteric plexus of the colon, which causes hypertonicity and obstruction.
- Involved area ranges in length from a short segment limited to the distal sigmoid and rectum (most common) to the entire colon.
- The male-to-female ratio is 4:1.
- Eighty percent of patients present with failure to pass meconium in the first 24 hours of life, intermittent diarrhea/obstruction.
- The diagnosis is made by rectal biopsy—aganglionosis always involves the anus and continues proximally.
- The treatment is surgical resection of the affected colon.
- If untreated, Hirschsprung disease can lead to toxic megacolon, enterocolitis, and sepsis.
- Contrast enema: Rectum less distensible than sigmoid (rectosigmoid ratio < 1); transition zone from an abnormally small distal colon to a dilated proximal portion. Denervated colon may be spasmodic.

✓ Pearls & ✗ Pitfalls

- ✓ The critical view on the contrast enema is the early-filling lateral view, demonstrating that the rectum is less distensible than the sigmoid and showing a transition zone.
- ✓ The affected portion always includes the anus and continues proximally.
- ✓ Of patients with Hirschsprung disease, 10 to 15% have Down syndrome.
- ✗ Enema should be administered without bowel preparation. Prior rectal manipulation can cause false-negative results.
- ✗ The transition zone may be subtle/absent during the first week of life.
- ✗ Total colonic Hirschsprung disease can appear as a microcolon.

Case 29

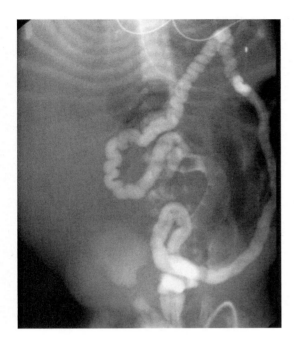

Clinical Presentation

A newborn with failure to pass meconium.

■ **Imaging Findings**

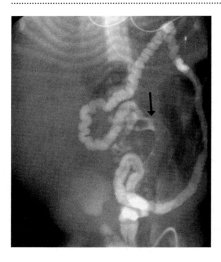

Contrast enema demonstrates a small, unused colon. Contrast refluxed into the terminal ileum outlines multiple small filling defects (*arrow*). There are dilated loops of small bowel more proximally.

■ **Differential Diagnosis**

- **Meconium ileus:** These findings are typical of meconium ileus.
- *Meconium plug syndrome:* Meconium plugs should be found throughout the colon, not solely in the terminal ileum. Usually, there is a transition point at the splenic flexure with dilated colon more proximally. Plugs may be passed during administration of the enema.
- *Ileal atresia:* This is not associated with meconium but does cause a blind-ending ileum; usually, multiple air-fluid levels are present.

■ **Essential Facts**

- Abnormally thick meconium obstructs the distal ileum.
- Signs and symptoms include failure to pass meconium and abdominal distension.
- Almost all patients with meconium ileus have cystic fibrosis (CF).
- Meconium ileus can lead to perforation and meconium peritonitis with stenosis/atresia or volvulus of a dilated segment.
- The treatment of uncomplicated meconium ileus is the serial administration of hyperosmotic, water-soluble enemas.
- The terminal ileum is packed with dried meconium pellets.
- Prenatal ultrasound: there are dilated, echogenic loops of bowel, particularly in the right lower quadrant.
- Plain radiographs: There are multiple dilated loops of bowel, sometimes with possibly bubbly lucencies in the right lower quadrant that mimic pneumatosis. No air-fluid levels are seen.

- Contrast enema: There is microcolon. Reflux of contrast into the terminal ileum shows the meconium pellets as small filling defects.
- Hyperosmolar contrast enema is also therapeutic, usually stimulating the passage of meconium.

■ **Other Imaging Findings**

- Ultrasound: there are dilated, thick-walled loops of bowel with hyperechoic contents.

✓ **Pearls & ✗ Pitfalls**

✓ Almost all patients with meconium ileus have CF. Fifteen percent of patients with CF present with meconium ileus.
✓ Meconium ileus causes the most severe microcolon.
✗ The concentration of water-soluble contrast to use for the enema is controversial. It should be somewhat hyperosmolar.

Case 30

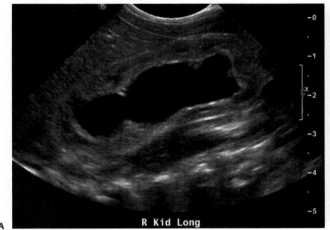

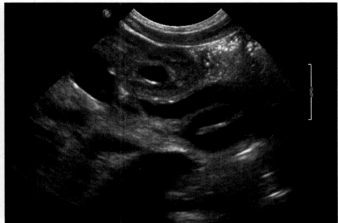

A

B

■ Clinical Presentation

A newborn with in utero hydronephrosis.

Further Work-up

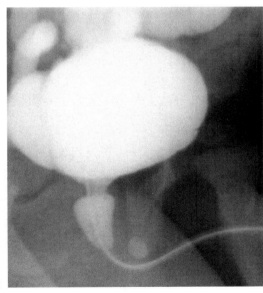

C

■ Imaging Findings

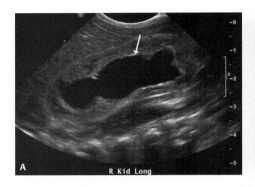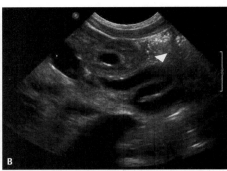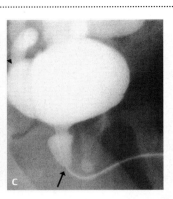

(A,B) Sonographic images demonstrate severe hydronephrosis (*arrow*) and hydro-ureter (*arrowhead*). The findings were present bilaterally. **(C)** Oblique image from a voiding cysto-urethrogram demonstrates a bullet-shaped dilatation of the posterior urethra (*arrow*) with reflux into the (*arrowhead*) dilated ureter. The more distal urethra is of normal caliber.

■ Differential Diagnosis

- **Posterior urethral valves:** Bilateral hydronephrosis with hydroureter suggests a bladder outlet obstruction. The posterior urethral dilatation is typical.
- *Ureterovesical junction obstruction:* The ultrasound findings are also consistent with this diagnosis, but the posterior urethra would not be dilated.
- *Vesicoureteral reflux (VUR):* Severe VUR can cause hydroureter and hydronephrosis, but not urethral dilatation.

■ Essential Facts

- A varying degree of urethral obstruction is due to fusion/prominence of the normal folds of the posterior urethra.
- Posterior urethral valves occur exclusively in males.
- The severity of the obstruction determines the age of the patient at presentation.
- The condition can cause oligohydramnios and pulmonary hypoplasia in utero. It may present later with urinary tract infection, poor urinary stream, hesitancy, and straining.
- Severe cases can lead to severe reflux nephropathy.
- The treatment is endoscopic valve ablation.
- Voiding cystourethrogram: There is a dilated posterior urethra, but actual valve tissue may not be seen. The bladder can be trabeculated and have diverticula. Patients almost always have VUR.
- Ultrasound: A thick bladder wall and dilated posterior urethra may be seen. Complications such as urinary ascites or urinoma may also be identified.

✓ Pearls & ✗ Pitfalls

- ✓ The hallmark is a dilated posterior urethra with an abrupt change to a more normal-caliber distal urethra.
- ✗ A urethral catheter left in place during voiding may obscure the change in caliber in the urethra.

Case 31

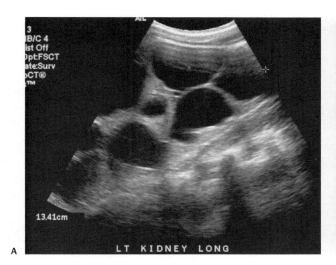

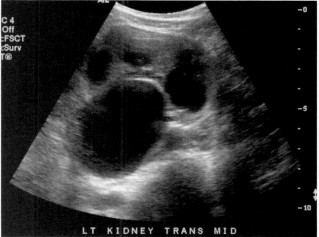

A — LT KIDNEY LONG   13.41cm

B — LT KIDNEY TRANS MID

■ Clinical Presentation

An infant with hydronephrosis on prenatal ultrasound.

Further Work-up

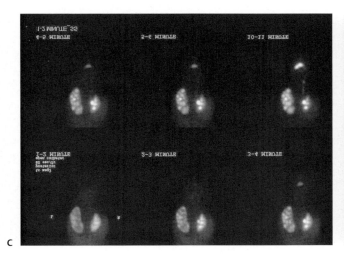

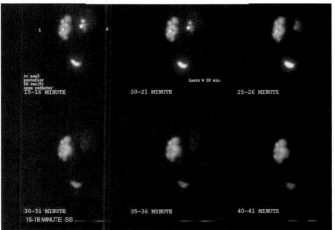

C

D

■ Imaging Findings

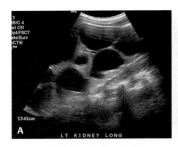
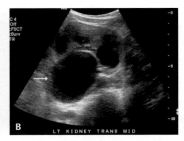
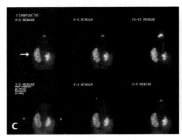
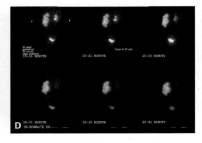

(A,B) Sonographic images of the left kidney demonstrate multiple ovoid, anechoic structures. Note the dilated central anechoic structure, consistent with a dilated renal pelvis (*arrow*), making this more likely to be hydronephrosis than multiple cysts. **(C,D)** Images from a MAG3 (mercapto-acetyl-triglycine) nuclear medicine study demonstrate the delayed uptake and excretion of radioactive tracer by the enlarged left kidney. Note the dilated calyces (*arrow*).

■ Differential Diagnosis

- ***Ureteropelvic junction (UPJ) obstruction:*** A hydronephrotic kidney without hydroureter but with delayed uptake and excretion of MAG3 is consistent with UPJ obstruction.
- *Multicystic dysplastic kidney (MCDK):* The ultrasound appearance can be consistent with MCDK, but an MCDK would not have MAG3 uptake.
- *Ureterovesical junction (UVJ) obstruction:* These findings can be consistent with UVJ obstruction, but the absence of hydroureter on sonography makes this less likely.

■ Essential Facts

- Multiple etiologic factors have been postulated, including abnormal smooth muscle, abnormal innervation, and crossing vessels.
- UPJ obstruction is more common on the left than the right.
- In the newborn, it is two times more common in boys.
- Signs and symptoms include prenatal hydronephrosis, infection, intermittent pain, and hematuria.
- Long-standing high-grade obstruction can lead to decreased renal function.
- UPJ obstructions may regress or deteriorate spontaneously.
- The treatment is pyeloplasty.
- Marked hydronephrosis ends sharply at the UPJ obstruction with no urethral dilatation.
- Nuclear medicine is used to follow the differential renal function and degree of obstruction.

✓ Pearls & ✗ Pitfalls

- ✓ UPJ obstruction is the most common form of urinary tract obstruction in children.
- ✓ Imaging of the kidneys within the first week of life can underestimate the degree of hydronephrosis because of dehydration. If the kidneys are normal on ultrasound within the first week of life, imaging should be repeated.
- ✗ Pelvocaliectasis can persist following successful pyeloplasty. Renal growth and drainage on nuclear studies confirm the success of surgery.

Case 32

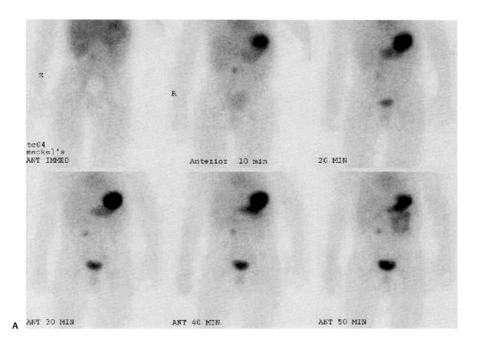

■ Clinical Presentation

A 4-year-old boy with recurrent episodes of abdominal pain and rectal bleeding.

Further Work-up

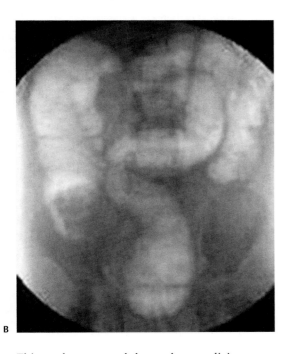

This study prompted the nuclear medicine scan.

■ Imaging Findings

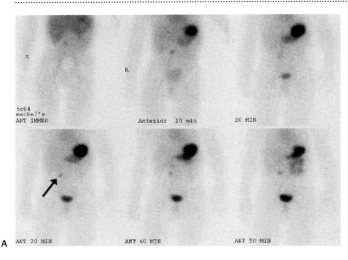
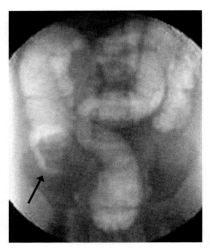

(A) Pertechnetate nuclear medicine scan demonstrates a focal accumulation of radioactive tracer in the right lower quadrant that is at least as intense as that in the stomach and increases over time (*arrow*). **(B)** Frontal view from an air-contrast enema demonstrates a mass within the cecum, consistent with intussusception (*arrow*).

■ Differential Diagnosis

- *Meckel diverticulum:* The pertechnetate scan is consistent with Meckel diverticulum. Meckel diverticula can act as lead points for intussusception.
- *Intestinal duplication containing gastric mucosa:* This is also seen in the right lower quadrant and could serve as a lead point for intussusception, but it is less common than Meckel diverticulum.
- *Inflammatory bowel disease or appendicitis:* May cause an early, mildly increased accumulation of pertechnetate due to hyperemia but would not cause intussusception.

■ Essential Facts

- Meckel diverticula are remnants of the omphalomesenteric duct, 50% of which contain gastric mucosa.
- Rule of 2s: 2% of population, within 2 feet of the ileocecal valve, 2 inches in length, clinical symptoms before the age of 2 years.
- Presentation/complications include pain, gastrointestinal bleeding, intussusception, and perforation.
- The treatment is surgical resection.
- Pertechnetate nuclear medicine scan: Accumulation in a Meckel diverticulum increases with time, similar to gastric activity. The diverticulum usually does not communicate with the bowel lumen, so the position of the activity does not change unless there is active bleeding.
- False-negative scans occur when the diverticulum does not contain gastric mucosa or when blood supply to the diverticulum is impaired.

■ Other Imaging Findings

- Computed tomography/ultrasound: Meckel diverticulum may be confused with appendicitis—inflamed, blind-ending pouch near the cecum.

✓ Pearls & ✗ Pitfalls

- ✓ Cimetidine, pentagastrin, and glucagon all increase the sensitivity of nuclear medicine imaging for the detection of Meckel diverticulum.
- ✗ Meckel diverticula can be difficult to diagnose if they do not contain gastric mucosa.

Case 33

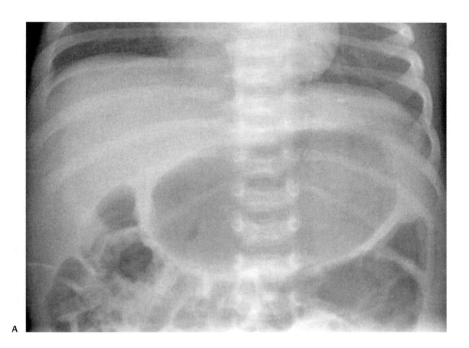

A

Clinical Presentation

A 1-month-old infant with vomiting.

Further Work-up

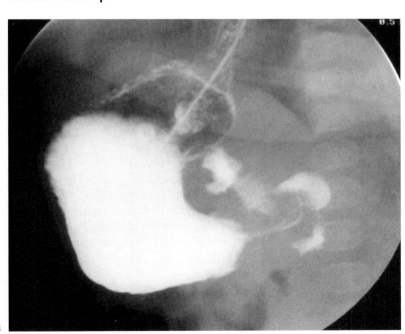

B

■ Imaging Findings

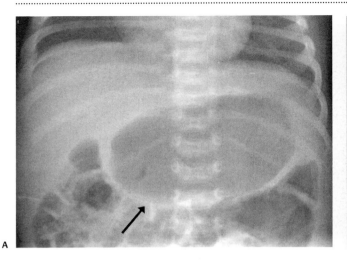 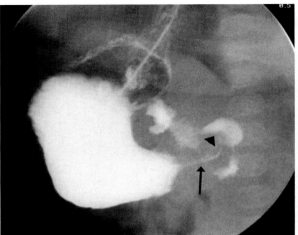

(A) Frontal abdominal radiograph demonstrates a markedly air-distended stomach (*arrow*) with air in the more distal portion of the gastrointestinal (GI) tract. **(B)** Barium upper GI image demonstrates a pyloric channel that is elongated and narrowed ("string sign," *arrow*). The thickened pyloric muscle impresses the duodenal bulb ("mushroom sign," *arrowhead*).

■ Differential Diagnosis

- **Hypertrophic pyloric stenosis:** The combination of a distended stomach with the string and mushroom signs on upper GI images is consistent with pyloric stenosis.
- *Annular pancreas:* The plain film findings support this, but annular pancreas narrows the duodenum below the bulb, not the pylorus.
- *Duodenal web:* The plain film findings support this, but the pylorus would be normal and the duodenum would be dilated.

■ Essential Facts

- Hypertrophic pyloric stenosis is an idiopathic hypertrophy of the pylorus that is gradually progressive and may spontaneously regress after many weeks.
- It presents with progressive nonbilious vomiting (eventually projectile) in a previously healthy infant.
- Physical examination reveals a palpable antral mass (called an "olive").
- It occurs at 2 to 12 weeks of age (or later if the patient was premature).
- It is four times more common in males.
- The treatment is pyloromyotomy.

■ Other Imaging Findings

- Fluoroscopy: May see exaggerated gastric motility ("caterpillar stomach"). The shoulders of the hypertrophic pylorus may indent the gastric antrum.
- Ultrasound: Abnormally thickened pyloric muscle and elongated channel. Normal measurements of the pylorus are debated; however, a single wall thickness of more than 3 to 4 mm and a pyloric length of more than 16 mm are commonly accepted as abnormal. Additionally, the echogenic mucosal layer may appear hypertrophic, and real-time imaging should demonstrate little to no passage of gastric contents through the pylorus, along with hyperperistalsis of the stomach.

✓ Pearls & ✗ Pitfalls

- ✓ In strongly suspected cases of pyloric stenosis, ultrasound is the test of choice.
- ✓ Pylorospasm may appear similar to pyloric stenosis, but the findings are transient.
- ✗ Hypertrophic pyloric stenosis develops progressively. Early findings may not support the diagnosis but will become clearer on subsequent examinations.

Case 34

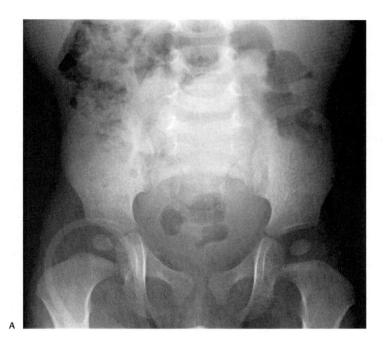

A

■ Clinical Presentation

A 2-year-old boy with a urinary tract infection. After completion of a course of antibiotics, abdominal pain, fever, and decreased urine output developed.

Further Work-up

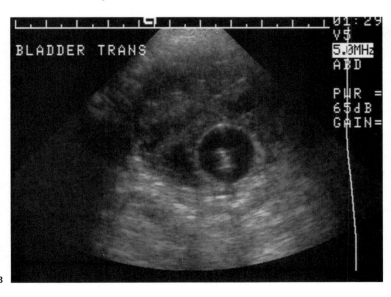

B

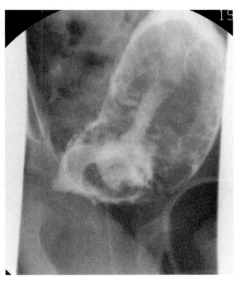

C

■ Imaging Findings

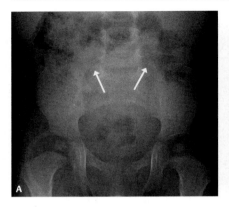 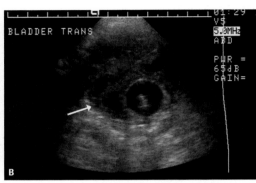 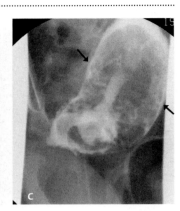

(A) Scout view from a voiding cystourethrogram (VCUG) demonstrates a soft-tissue mass in the pelvis that is displacing bowel loops superiorly (*arrows*). **(B)** Transverse sonogram of the urinary bladder demonstrates an intraluminal mass around the Foley catheter balloon (*arrow*). **(C)** Oblique image from the VCUG demonstrates a large, irregular filling defect in the distended bladder lumen (*arrows*).

■ Differential Diagnosis

- **Rhabdomyosarcoma:** A large bladder mass in a child is consistent with rhabdomyosarcoma.
- *Bladder hematoma:* Although a bladder hematoma could have this appearance, it would be unlikely without a history of significant trauma or chemotherapy.
- *Hematometrocolpos:* This can present as a pelvic mass and appear echogenic on sonography, but the mass would not be in the bladder surrounding the Foley catheter.

■ Essential Facts

- Rhabdomyosarcoma is a small, round blue cell tumor.
- It may originate anywhere in the body, but the head/neck is the most common site.
- In the pelvis, it may originate from the bladder, vagina, uterus, prostate, or paratesticular tissues.
- It may metastasize to lung, liver, and bone.
- The peak age is 2 to 5 years.
- Genitourinary rhabdomyosarcoma is two to three times more common in males. Rhabdomyosarcoma of the head, neck, or extremities exhibits no gender predilection.
- Treatment includes surgery, chemotherapy, and radiation.
- The prognosis is worse if the tumor occurs in the 1st year of life.
- Rhabdomyosarcomas are typically large cystic or solid tumors with a significant mass effect.

■ Other Imaging Findings

- Computed tomography: There is a heterogeneously enhancing mass. Look for local invasion, adjacent adenopathy, and lung or liver metastases.

✓ Pearls & ✗ Pitfalls

- ✓ The botryoid subtype often presents as a polypoid mass resembling a cluster of grapes and protruding from the vagina.
- ✓ The prostate is the most frequent site of pelvic origin in boys.
- ✗ This is the most common neoplasm of the lower urinary tract.

Case 35

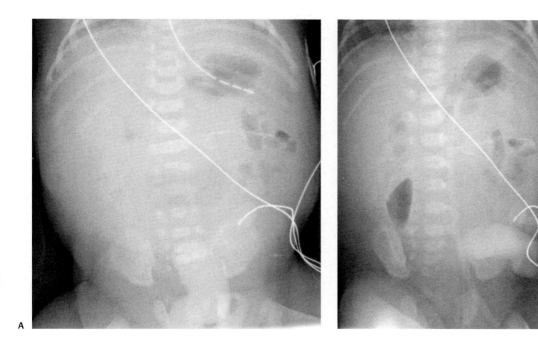

A

B

■ Clinical Presentation

A neonate with failure to pass meconium.

Further Work-up

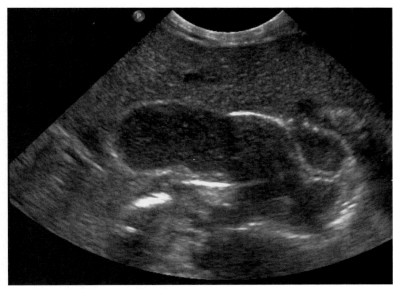

C

◼ Imaging Findings

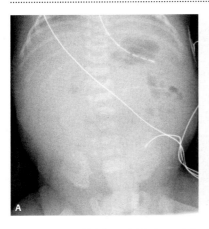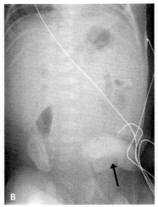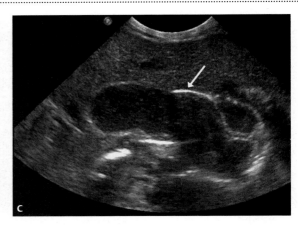

(A,B) Supine and left lateral decubitus abdominal radiographs demonstrate subtle curvilinear calcifications in the midabdomen, with a paucity of distal bowel gas. Note the appearance of the umbilical cord as a soft-tissue mass superimposed over the left lower quadrant (*arrow*). **(C)** Sonogram of the midabdomen demonstrates a well-defined ovoid hypoechoic mass with hyperechoic walls (*arrow*).

◼ Differential Diagnosis

- ***Meconium pseudocyst:*** Curvilinear calcifications in the abdomen of a newborn who has failed to pass meconium suggest in utero perforation from meconium ileus leading to pseudocyst formation.
- *Neuroblastoma:* Although 30% of neuroblastomas have radiographically detectable calcifications, the calcifications are generally chunkier and not limited to the edge of the mass.
- *Gastrointestinal duplication cyst:* Although calcification is occasionally seen in the cyst wall, the findings here lack the sonographic "gut signature" (echogenic mucosa, hypoechoic muscular layer, and echogenic serosa).

◼ Essential Facts

- In utero intestinal perforation leads to the peritoneal leakage of meconium, which becomes walled off.
- The timing of the perforation is typically at 4 to 9 months' gestation.
- Treatment is surgical.
- Intestinal obstruction is not always present because the perforation may heal in utero and the bowel may recanalize.
- Plain radiographs: soft-tissue mass, abdominal calcifications, dilated bowel loops.
- Ultrasound: heterogeneous mass with echogenic (calcified) walls.

✓ Pearls & ✗ Pitfalls

- ✓ Calcifications become visible within a week of perforation.
- ✓ Calcifications follow the contour of the peritoneum and can extend into the scrotum as the consequence of inguinal hernia.
- ✗ It is necessary to search for causes of the perforation: meconium ileus, intestinal obstruction, or in utero volvulus.

Case 36

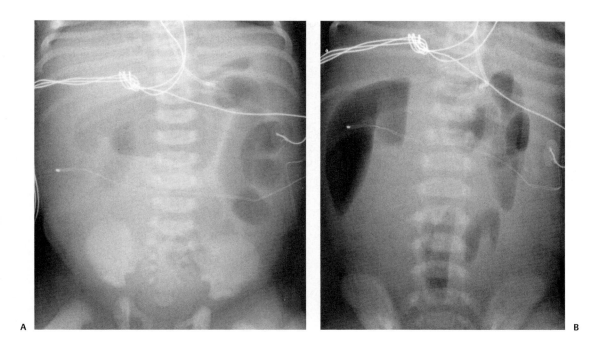

A

B

Clinical Presentation

A neonate with vomiting and abdominal distension.

Further Work-up

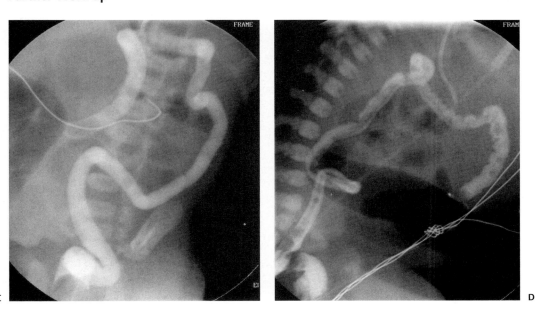

C

D

■ Imaging Findings

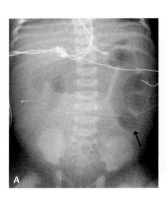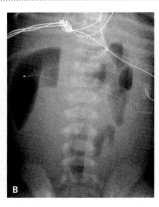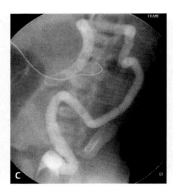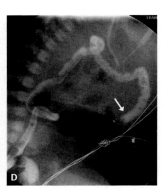

(A,B) Abdominal plain films show multiple loops of dilated small bowel with air-fluid levels. There is no air distally (*arrow*). **(C,D)** Contrast enema: The entire colon is small and unused. Contrast does not reflux into the terminal ileum (*arrow*).

■ Differential Diagnosis

- **Ileal atresia:** Findings of microcolon and the inability to reflux contrast into the terminal ileum suggest ileal atresia.
- *Meconium ileus:* Contrast should reflux into the terminal ileum to outline obstructing meconium pellets.
- *Total colonic Hirschsprung disease:* Can be difficult to differentiate. May see a transition zone and should be able to reflux contrast into terminal ileum.

■ Essential Facts

- An in utero vascular accident in which the devascularized bowel becomes necrotic results in atresia.
- Patients most commonly present with a distended abdomen and failure to pass meconium.
- The treatment is surgical resection.
- The prognosis depends on the amount of normal bowel.
- Complications include short-gut syndrome, dysmotility, and functional obstruction.
- Plain radiography: dilated loops of small bowel with air-fluid levels
- If distal obstruction is suspected and there are no signs of perforation, a water-soluble contrast enema should be administered to confirm the diagnosis.

■ Other Imaging Findings

- Prenatal ultrasound: echogenic, dilated loops of bowel

✓ Pearls & ✗ Pitfalls

- ✓ The earlier in gestation the obstruction occurs, the smaller the caliber of the colon.
- ✓ On plain film, the finding of meconium peritonitis with small-bowel obstruction is virtually pathognomonic for small-bowel atresia.
- ✗ Ileal atresia can be difficult to differentiate from total colonic Hirschsprung disease. Suction biopsy may be required.
- ✗ The differentiation between jejunal and ileal atresia by imaging is not clinically important because multiple atresias can occur and the surgeon will evaluate the entire small bowel regardless of the imaging findings.

Case 37

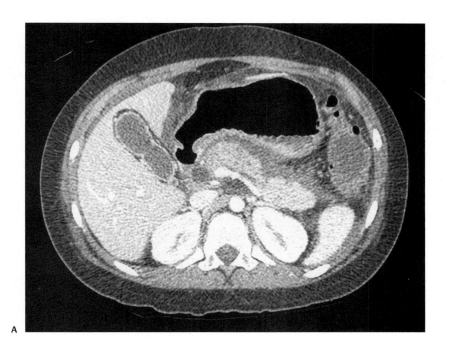

A

■ Clinical Presentation

A 10-year-old girl with abdominal pain.

Further Work-up

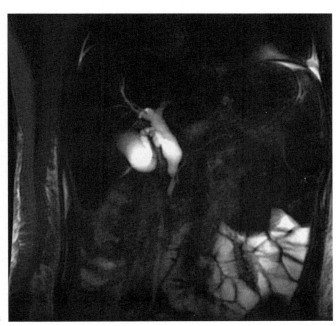

B

■ Imaging Findings

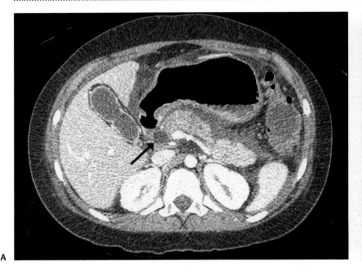 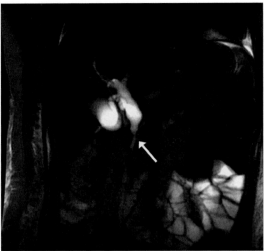

(A) Axial computed tomography image: There is fluid around the pancreas, and the distal common bile duct (CBD) is dilated (*arrow*). **(B)** Magnetic resonance cholangiopancreatography (MRCP): There is diffuse dilatation of the extrahepatic bile duct. Note the insertion of the pancreatic duct onto the CBD proximal to the papilla (long common channel, *arrow*).

■ Differential Diagnosis

- **Choledochal cyst:** Marked dilatation of the CBD associated with a long common channel of the pancreatic duct and CBD is consistent with choledochal cyst.
- *Stricture of the CBD:* Although this can cause dilatation of the CBD, it would not explain the long common channel or the pancreatitis.
- *Obstructing stone/mass:* From the single computed tomography image, this would be high on the differential diagnosis list, but no stone or mass is seen. Additionally, the MRCP does not show filling defects or irregularity of the ducts to suggest stones or a mass.

■ Essential Facts

- A possible etiology is a long common channel of the pancreatic duct and CBD that allows mixing of the pancreatic and biliary enzymes. This weakens and dilates the CBD and can lead to pancreatitis.
- The Todani classification describes at least five different types of choledochal cyst, differentiated by the portions of the ducts that are dilated.
- The most common presenting signs and symptoms in infants include prolonged cholestasis/jaundice, hepatomegaly, and mass. Older patients typically present with recurrent cholangitis and pancreatitis.
- Choledochal cysts are more common in females (female-to-male ratio, 3:1–4:1) and in the Far East.
- The treatment is complete surgical excision.
- Complications: increased risk for adenocarcinoma, stone formation, bile duct perforation, cholangitis, pancreatitis, cirrhosis

- Choledochal cysts comprise a spectrum of abnormalities involving saccular or fusiform dilatation of the intrahepatic and/or extrahepatic bile ducts, as well as a long common channel of the pancreatic duct and CBD.
- Magnetic resonance imaging/MRCP: Demonstrates the pancreatic duct and CBD and can be helpful to demonstrate the long common channel.

■ Other Imaging Findings

- Ultrasound, transhepatic cholangiogram, and ERCP all demonstrate biliary duct dilatation or outpouching.

✓ Pearls & ✗ Pitfalls

- ✓ A CBD measuring more than 10 mm in a child strongly suggests a choledochal cyst.
- ✗ A Todani type V choledochal cyst is Caroli disease (cavernous ectasia of the intrahepatic ducts). It is controversial whether Caroli disease is actually a type of choledochal cyst.

Case 38

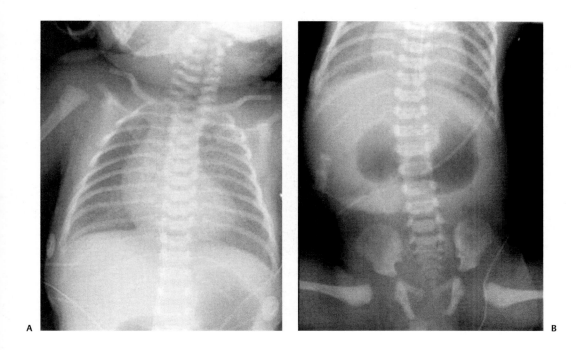

A

B

▓ Clinical Presentation

A neonate with persistent vomiting.

■ Imaging Findings

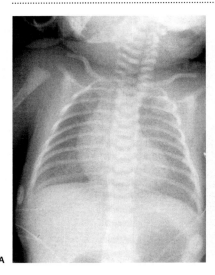
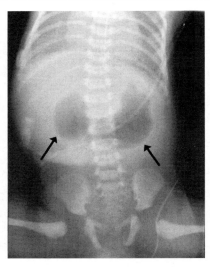

(A,B) Frontal chest and abdominal radiographs demonstrate gaseous dilatation of the stomach and duodenum with no gas distal to this point in the gastrointestinal tract, a pattern that is often referred to as a "double bubble" (*arrows*).

■ Differential Diagnosis

- **Duodenal atresia:** The findings of a dilated stomach and duodenum with a complete absence of distal bowel gas are classic for duodenal atresia.
- *Malrotation with midgut volvulus:* Once volvulus occurs, malrotation can also present with complete duodenal obstruction. However, this is typically an acute event, and the duodenum will not be dilated to the same extent as in duodenal atresia.
- *Duodenal web:* A duodenal web can also cause duodenal dilatation, but the obstruction is not complete, and as a result, patients often present later and distal bowel gas is present.

■ Essential Facts

- In many patients, duodenal atresia is diagnosed by prenatal sonography, which shows polyhydramnios and a double bubble of fluid-filled, dilated stomach and duodenum.
- Patients present in first 24 hours of life with bilious vomiting.
- Most cases are thought to result from failure of recanalization of the duodenum after the endodermal proliferation that occurs at approximately the 8th week of gestation.
- The duodenum is the most common site of gastrointestinal tract atresia.
- Approximately one-half of patients have associated anomalies such as Down syndrome (30%), annular pancreas, and malrotation.
- Surgical correction is required to sustain life.

✓ Pearls & ✗ Pitfalls

- ✓ There is no need to perform an upper gastrointestinal examination if the clinical and plain radiographic findings are typical.
- ✓ Further imaging to distinguish between causes of high-grade congenital duodenal obstruction is unnecessary because surgery is required in any case.
- ✓ Look for associated findings, such as esophageal atresia, congenital heart disease, and 11 pairs of ribs.

Case 39

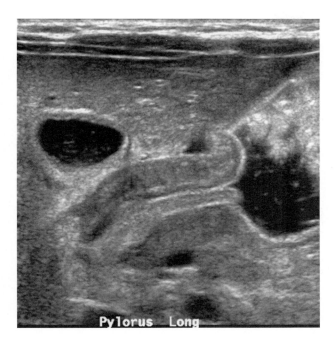

■ Clinical Presentation

A 4-week-old infant with projectile vomiting.

■ **Imaging Findings**

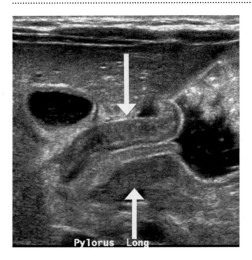

Pylorus Long

A longitudinal sonogram of the pyloric region demonstrates a fluid-distended stomach and a markedly elongated and thickened pylorus (*arrows*). During 10 minutes of sonographic monitoring, no emptying of the gastric contents through the pylorus was observed.

■ **Differential Diagnosis**

- *Hypertrophic pyloric stenosis:* A persistently elongated and thickened pyloric channel is typical of this disorder.
- *Pylorospasm:* The pylorus can appear elongated and thickened, but this appearance is transient, and antegrade emptying of the gastric contents will occur when the pylorus relaxes.
- *Gastroesophageal reflux:* Most infants with nonbilious vomiting demonstrate no anatomic abnormality, and sonographic examination of the pylorus will reveal no elongation or thickening.

■ **Essential Facts**

- Hypertrophic pyloric stenosis usually presents between 2 weeks and 2 months of age.
- The male-to-female ratio is 4:1.
- This is an acquired (not congenital) lesion in infants who previously fed well.
- Most patients are immediately hungry after they vomit, unlike patients with infectious causes of vomiting.
- A hypertrophic pylorus may be palpable as an "olive" just beneath the abdominal wall.
- Precise quantitative diagnostic criteria are difficult to provide, but in general, the length of the pyloric channel is more than 16 mm and the total diameter of the pyloric channel is more than 15 mm.

■ **Other Imaging Findings**

- Barium upper gastrointestinal imaging demonstrates a pyloric indentation on the distal antrum ("shouldering") and an elongated, narrowed pyloric channel ("string sign").

✓ **Pearls & ✗ Pitfalls**

- ✓ The classic clinical picture is dehydration and hypochloremic metabolic alkalosis.
- ✓ This is the most common reason for laparoscopy/laparotomy in patients younger than 1 year of age.
- ✓ Hypertrophic pyloric stenosis is not a "middle of the night" emergency; surgery is usually performed the next day.
- ✓ Contrary to what is stated in many textbooks, the condition is probably not substantially more common in first-born infants.
- ✓ Whether imaging is by sonography or barium upper gastrointestinal study, the pyloric channel should be observed over time to ensure that it does not relax and open up.

Case 40

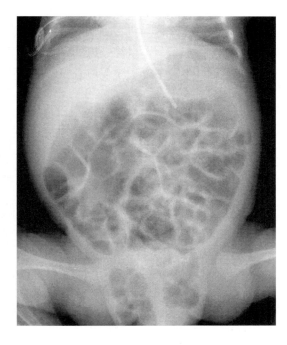

■ Clinical Presentation

An irritable infant with bilious vomiting.

■ Imaging Findings

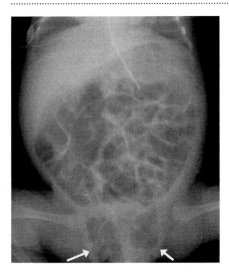

An abdominal radiograph demonstrates a large amount of abnormally dilated bowel throughout the abdomen, suspected of being a distal bowel obstruction. Moreover, gas-containing, dilated bowel is seen in the scrotum (*arrows*), consistent with bilateral herniation of the bowel through the inguinal canals.

■ Differential Diagnosis

- ***Mechanical bowel obstruction:*** In this case, the plain radiographic findings are essentially diagnostic of bilateral inguinal hernias, which are almost certainly the cause of the patient's obstructive symptoms.
- *Malrotation with midgut volvulus:* In any infant with bilious vomiting, malrotation is the diagnosis to exclude. In this case, the finding of bowel in the scrotum is key, but many patients with a hernia may not have gas in the scrotum or inguinal canal, and a barium upper gastrointestinal examination may be warranted to rule out malrotation.
- *Functional ileus:* Many patients with vomiting and abdominal distension have nonanatomic conditions, such as infectious enterocolitis and formula intolerance. In such cases, there may be diffuse dilatation of the bowel, but gas should be present in the rectum, with no identifiable nondilated bowel.

■ Essential Facts

- Acquired causes of acute intestinal obstruction in infants include intussusception, incarcerated hernia, malrotation with midgut volvulus, postoperative adhesions, and stricture secondary to necrotizing enterocolitis.
- Inguinal hernias are approximately four times more common in males than in females.
- The incidence is 10 times higher in premature infants than in full-term infants and varies directly with the degree of prematurity. Most patients present in the first month of life.
- The condition is related to a patent processus vaginalis.

✓ Pearls & ✘ Pitfalls

- ✓ When a scrotal mass is present, sonography is generally the examination of choice.
- ✓ The term *incarceration* implies that the hernia sac cannot be reduced back into the peritoneal cavity.
- ✓ In children, the most common cause of direct inguinal hernia is repair of any indirect inguinal hernia.
- ✓ Umbilical hernias rarely become incarcerated, and most resolve spontaneously in the first few years of life.

Case 41

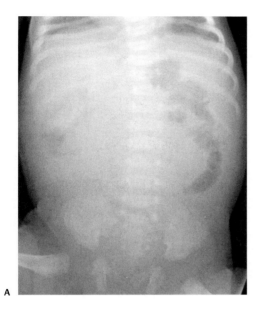

A

■ Clinical Presentation

A neonate with irritability, poor feeding, and bilious vomiting.

Further Work-up

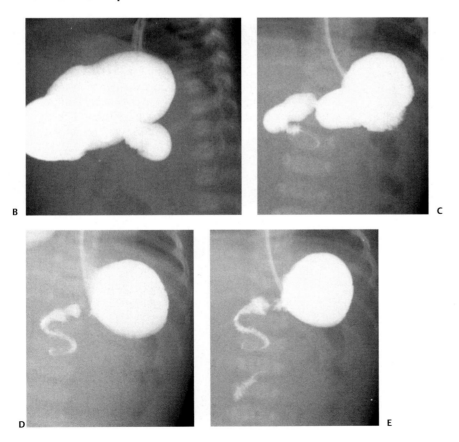

B

C

D

E

■ Imaging Findings

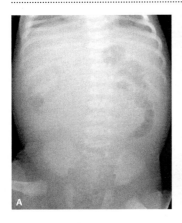
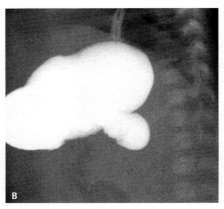
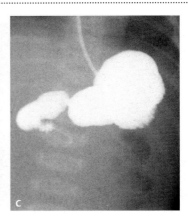
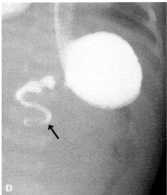
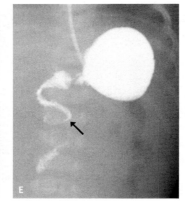

(A) An abdominal radiograph demonstrates a paucity of bowel gas in the central abdomen, but no clear evidence of obstruction. This is an abnormal but nonspecific pattern of bowel gas. **(B–E)** Four images from a barium upper gastrointestinal examination performed with an orogastric tube. **(B)** Image demonstrates what could be mistaken for a complete duodenal obstruction, although the degree of dilatation is insufficient to suggest a congenital atresia or high-grade stenosis. **(C)** Image demonstrates contrast material passing beyond this point. **(D,E)** Images demonstrate a classic "corkscrew" duodenum (*arrows*), secondary to midgut volvulus. Note that the duodenojejunal junction is positioned inferiorly and superimposed over the spine, indicating malrotation (*arrows*).

■ Differential Diagnosis

- ***Malrotation with midgut volvulus:*** The abnormally positioned duodenojejunal junction and the corkscrew or helical appearance of the duodenum are diagnostic of malrotation with midgut volvulus.
- ***"Wandering" duodenum:*** Particularly in small children, the duodenum may exhibit a somewhat irregular course, but such patients should have no obstruction and a normally positioned duodenojejunal junction.
- *Congenital duodenal obstruction:* Duodenal atresia presents within hours, but duodenal stenoses, including webs, often present later with bilious vomiting. In such cases, the proximal duodenum should be more dilated than in the acute obstruction of midgut volvulus, and the site of the obstruction should be easily identifiable.

■ Essential Facts

- The estimated incidence of malrotation is approximately 1 in 500.
- In 50% of patients with malrotation, it is diagnosed by 1 month of age, and in 75% by 1 year.
- Volvulus is secondary to a short mesenteric attachment of the gut to the posterior abdominal wall, which allows twisting.

- Normal attachment: The duodenojejunal junction is fixed by the ligament of Treitz in the left upper quadrant, the cecum in the right lower quadrant.
- Ladd bands are congenital adhesions found in patients with malrotation, which may cause duodenal obstruction.
- A dreaded complication of volvulus is ischemia/infarction of the bowel, which can result in sepsis and death, with long-term complications of stricture and short-gut syndrome among survivors.

✓ Pearls & ✗ Pitfalls

- ✓ Suspected midgut volvulus is a radiologic emergency.
- ✓ Malrotation is present in nearly all patients with congenital diaphragmatic hernia, gastroschisis, and omphalocele.
- ✓ The cecum is malpositioned in most—but not all—patients with malrotation, so a normal enema does not exclude the diagnosis.
- ✓ Cross-sectional imaging may show an abnormal relationship between the superior mesenteric artery (SMA) and superior mesenteric vein (SMV).
- ✓ Normally, the SMV is anterior and to the right of the SMA.
- ✗ Plain radiography does not exclude malrotation or volvulus, and findings may be normal.

Case 42

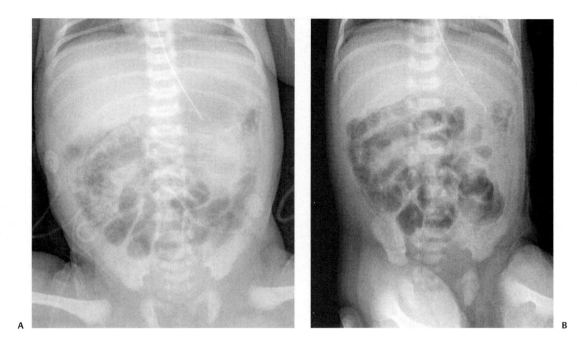

A   B

■ Clinical Presentation

A premature patient in the neonatal intensive care unit with gastric retention of feedings, abdominal distension, tachycardia, and tachypnea.

■ Imaging Findings

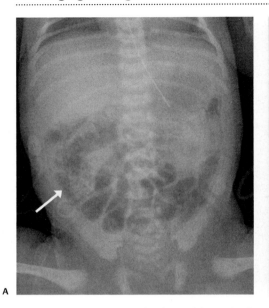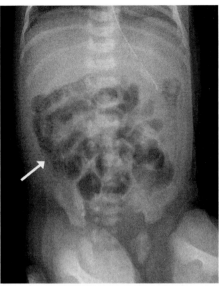

A

B

(A,B) Frontal and left lateral decubitus abdominal radiographs demonstrate a markedly abnormal pattern of bowel gas, with multiple segments of distended bowel and bubbly and linear lucencies most prominent on the right side (*arrows*). There is no evidence of pneumoperitoneum.

■ Differential Diagnosis

- ***Necrotizing enterocolitis (NEC):*** The bubbly and linear lucencies superimposed over the bowel gas are typical for pneumatosis intestinalis, a nearly diagnostic sign in this clinical setting.
- *Bowel obstruction:* Causes of neonatal bowel obstruction include malrotation with midgut volvulus and Hirschsprung disease, although the former should be associated with bilious vomiting and the latter with persistent stooling problems.
- *Functional ileus:* Often the consequence of systemic disease such as congenital heart disease or sepsis, infectious enterocolitis, or milk intolerance. The first two conditions can produce a picture very similar to that of NEC.

■ Essential Facts

- NEC is most common in premature infants; the incidence varies with the degree of prematurity.
- It presents with abdominal distension, bloody stools, feeding intolerance, gastric residuals, and systemic symptoms and signs.
- It is thought to be due to gut prematurity and a combination of intestinal ischemia and infection; hence it is treated by withholding feedings and antibiotics.
- Complications include death from perforation and sepsis, short-gut syndrome after bowel resection, and the later development of strictures.

- Decubitus or cross-table lateral radiographs are important to detect pneumoperitoneum, which is an indication for surgical intervention.
- Signs of pneumoperitoneum on supine radiographs include visualization of the falciform ligament and an ill-defined lucency over the epigastric region.
- Another important plain radiographic finding is gas within the portal venous system.
- Later, small-bowel and enema studies may be indicated to detect strictures in patients with signs of obstruction.

■ Other Imaging Findings

- Sonography can demonstrate bowel wall thickening as well as ascites and portal venous gas.

✓ Pearls & ✗ Pitfalls

- ✓ As more premature babies survive, the incidence of NEC has been increasing.
- ✓ Low-osmolar contrast studies of the bowel may demonstrate perforation, with the frank extravasation of contrast into the peritoneal cavity or the appearance of contrast in the urinary tract, meaning that it has leaked from the bowel and been absorbed by the peritoneal membrane.

Case 43

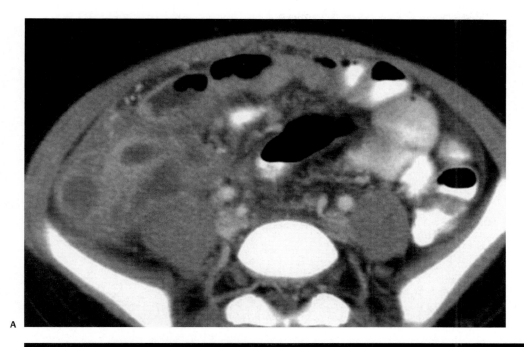

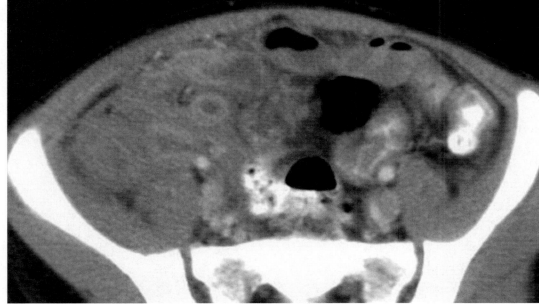

■ Clinical Presentation

A 7-year-old child with right lower quadrant abdominal pain and tenderness, low-grade fever, and anorexia.

■ Imaging Findings

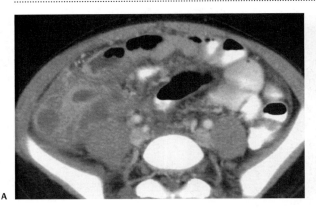
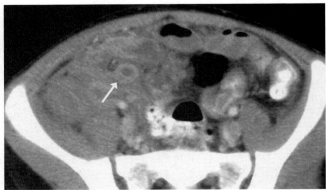

A   B

(A,B) Two axial computed tomography (CT) images after the oral and intravenous administration of contrast demonstrate inflammatory changes in the right lower quadrant with a dilated, fluid-filled tubular structure that has a thickened and enhancing wall (*arrow*).

■ Differential Diagnosis

- ***Appendicitis:*** The finding of a dilated appendix with wall thickening, increased enhancement, and surrounding inflammation is typical.
- *Mesenteric adenitis:* A nonsurgical condition associated with inflammation and/or infection of mesenteric lymph nodes, which are often clustered in the right lower quadrant. The appendix itself should appear normal.
- *Meckel diverticulum:* May be associated with right lower quadrant pain, but bleeding is a more frequently associated symptom than fever.

■ Essential Facts

- Appendicitis is the most common cause of urgent abdominal surgery in pediatric patients.
- The presenting symptoms and signs can be vague in young patients, leading to a delayed diagnosis and higher rate of perforation.
- It is secondary to obstruction of the appendiceal lumen by adenopathy or appendicolith, with resultant bacterial overgrowth, distension, and ischemia.

■ Other Imaging Findings

- Plain radiographs may demonstrate a right lower quadrant paucity of bowel gas or a soft-tissue mass, small-bowel obstruction, or appendicolith in up to 10% of cases.
- Sonography with a graded-compression technique may demonstrate the inflamed appendix as a noncompressible, hyperemic tubular structure. Patients often exhibit focal tenderness to palpation with the transducer. Sonography may also demonstrate an appendicolith as an echogenic, shadowing focus.

✓ Pearls & ✗ Pitfalls

- ✓ Appendicitis is rare in infants.
- ✓ Perforation can result in complications such as abscess formation, peritonitis, and sepsis.
- ✓ Imaging is frequently needed to assess postoperative patients with pain, tenderness, fever, and leukocytosis and look for abscesses.
- ✓ Radiologists differ over whether CT or sonography should serve as the first-line imaging examination.

Case 44

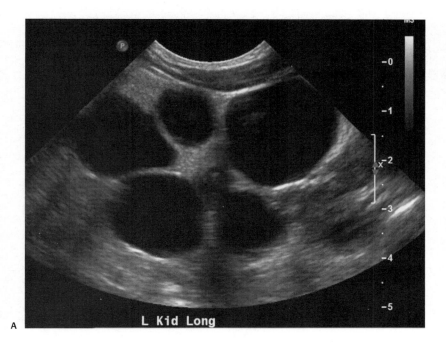

A

▣ Clinical Presentation

A newborn with a cystic mass seen on prenatal ultrasound.

Further Work-up

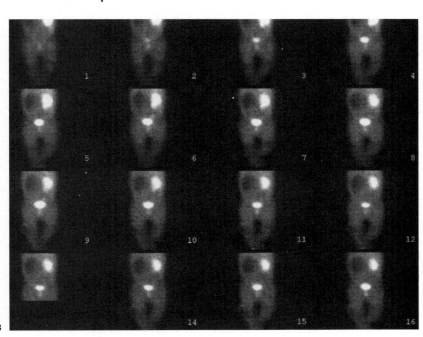

B

■ Imaging Findings

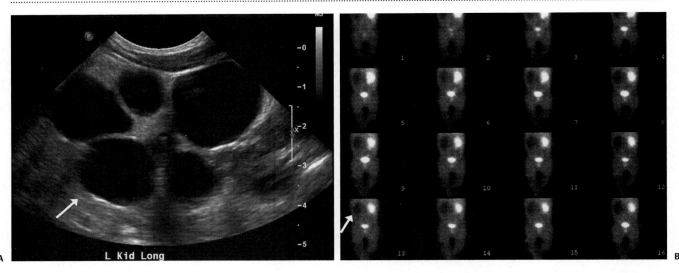

(A) Longitudinal sonogram: There are multiple cystic structures in the kidney that do not communicate (*arrow*). Normal renal cortex is not visualized. (B) MAG3 (mercapto-acetyl-triglycine) nuclear medicine scan: There is no uptake or excretion in the left kidney (*arrow*).

■ Differential Diagnosis

- ***Multicystic dysplastic kidney (MCDK):*** The finding of multiple discrete, noncommunicating cysts in a kidney demonstrating no function is consistent with MCDK.
- *Hydronephrosis:* This would appear as communicating cysts. A hydronephrotic kidney would show some function.
- *Wilms tumor:* Although Wilms tumor can appear cystic, some function should be demonstrated on MAG3 examination. Wilms tumor tends to occur in children aged 2 to 5 years.

■ Essential Facts

- MCDK is likely due to ureteral atresia or ureteropelvic junction obstruction in utero.
- It is typically discovered prenatally or in infancy as a palpable mass.
- Approximately half of cases show complete involution by age 7.
- Serial sonograms are used to monitor for involution and for complications such as focal enlargement (concern for Wilms), recurrent infection, mass effect, and hypertension.
- The treatment is resection only in complicated cases.
- The nonfunctioning kidney is replaced by numerous noncommunicating cysts of various sizes without normal intervening renal parenchyma.

■ Other Imaging Findings

- Ultrasound: The largest cyst is generally not in a central location, as it would be in hydronephrosis.
- On serial ultrasound examinations, the cysts should shrink, and the kidney will lose its reniform shape. Eventually, the kidney will not be detectable.
- Computed tomography: There is minimal to no enhancement with no excretion.

✓ Pearls & ✗ Pitfalls

- ✓ Always image the contralateral kidney to rule out pathology; 40% of cases have contralateral abnormalities.
- ✗ Can be segmental in duplicated kidneys
- ✗ Do not mistake MCDK for a multilocular cystic nephroma, which usually does not involve the entire kidney.

Case 45

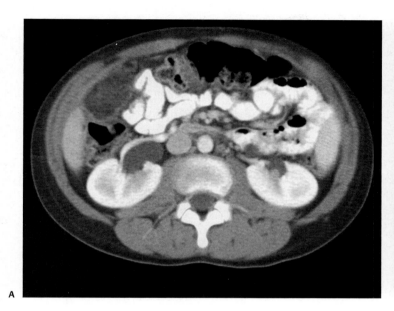
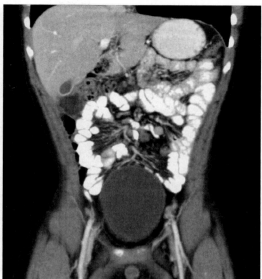

A

B

Clinical Presentation

A 12-year-old with right lower quadrant pain and fever.

■ Imaging Findings

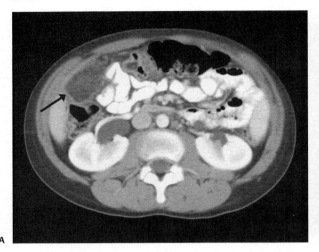 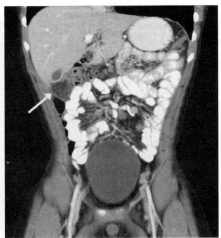

A   B

(A,B) Axial and coronal reformat computed tomography images after oral and intravenous administration of contrast demonstrate a heterogeneous mass to the right of the inferior tip of the liver and below the gallbladder containing both fat and streaky soft-tissue density *(arrows)*.

■ Differential Diagnosis

- **Omental infarction:** The finding of inflammatory stranding within a focal area of omental swelling is typical of this condition.
- *Appendicitis:* Also causes inflammatory stranding of fat, but this should be periappendiceal in location and associated with inflammatory changes in the appendix itself.
- *Epiploic appendagitis:* Also involves inflammation in the fat but is typically accompanied by a hyperattenuating ring.

■ Essential Facts

- Omental infarction is more common in boys than girls (male-to-female ratio, 3:1).
- Typically, the involved omentum is in the right lower quadrant, where it is most mobile and contains the most fat.
- Risk factors include obesity, strenuous activity, and abdominal trauma.
- It is often located anterior to the ascending or transverse colon.
- Surgery is not indicated if the diagnosis can be established preoperatively.

■ Other Imaging Findings

- Plain radiographs are usually negative.
- Sonography may demonstrate a hyperechoic mass just below the abdominal wall.

✓ Pearls & ✗ Pitfalls

- ✓ The presence of a hyperattenuating ring distinguishes epiploic appendagitis from omental infarction.
- ✓ In contrast to appendicitis, omental infarction and epiploic appendagitis are nonsurgical conditions.

Case 46

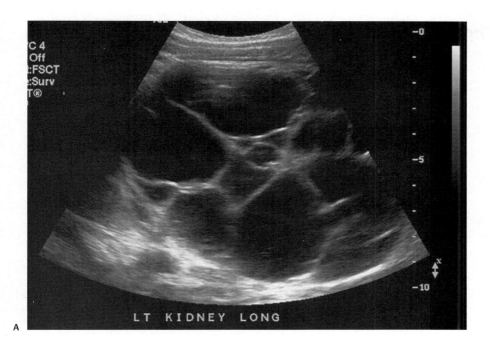

A

■ Clinical Presentation

A 6-month-old boy with a palpable abdominal mass.

Further Work-up

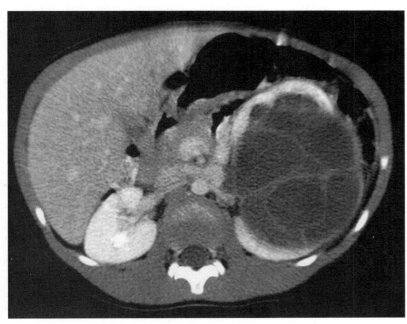

B

■ Imaging Findings

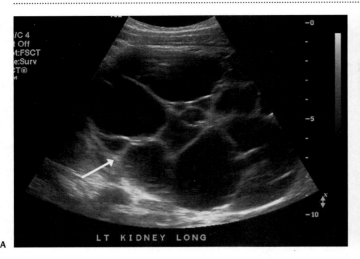
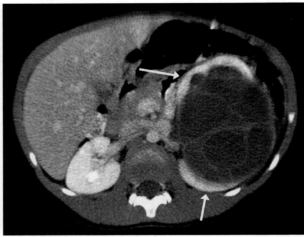

(A) Longitudinal ultrasound image: There is a multicystic mass in the left kidney (*arrow*). The cysts do not appear to communicate. **(B)** Contrast-enhanced computed tomography (CT) image: There is a multiloculate, fluid-density mass herniating into the left renal collecting system. Normally enhancing kidney surrounds it (*arrows*).

■ Differential Diagnosis

- **Multilocular cystic nephroma (MLCN):** A mass consisting of noncommunicating cysts that replaces only a portion of the kidney is consistent with MLCN.
- *Cystic Wilms tumor:* This can be difficult to differentiate, but Wilms tumor may invade the inferior vena cava.
- *Multicystic dysplastic kidney (MCDK):* There should be no functioning renal tissue on the CT image. MCDK usually involves the entire kidney rather than just a portion of it.

■ Essential Facts

- MLCN is a rare, nonhereditary benign neoplasm.
- The age/sex distribution is biphasic; MLCN is more common in infant/toddler boys and in women older than 40 years of age.
- The treatment is complete or partial nephrectomy.
- Local recurrence is possible.
- A large, multilocular cystic renal mass with a thick fibrous capsule may herniate into the renal pelvis; the septa and capsule may enhance.
- Portions of the mass may appear solid because of the presence of multiple tiny cysts.
- CT: May have calcification

■ Other Imaging Findings

- Magnetic resonance imaging: Signal may vary because of blood or protein in cyst fluid.

✓ Pearls & ✗ Pitfalls

- ✓ MLCN is not common in newborns/neonates.
- ✗ In a duplicated collecting system, MDCK of a single pole can look like MLCN.

Case 47

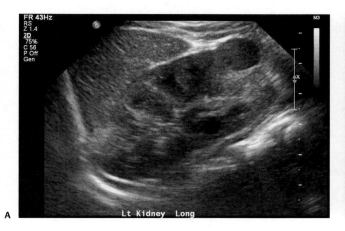
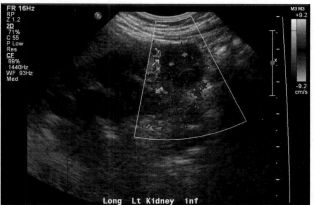

Clinical Presentation

A 3-year-old boy undergoing ultrasound for abdominal pain.

Further Work-up

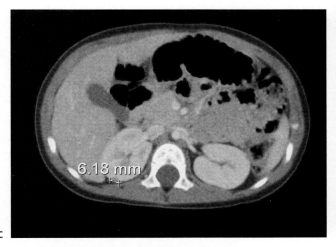
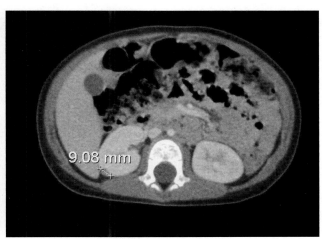

■ Imaging Findings

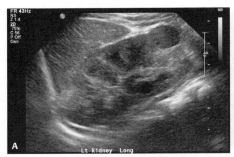
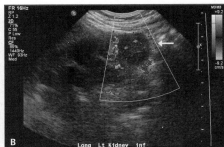
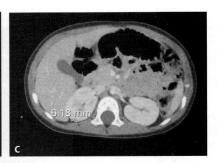
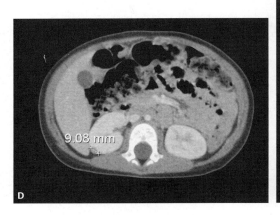
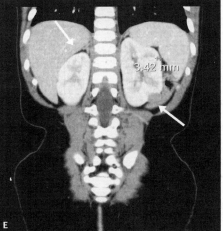

(A,B) US: There is a hypoechoic round mass at the lower pole of the left kidney with internal blood flow (*arrow*). **(C–E)** Computed tomography (CT): There are small, homogeneous, low-density nodules in the periphery of the kidneys (*arrows*). They do not enhance as strongly as the normal renal cortex.

■ Differential Diagnosis

- ***Nephroblastomatosis:*** Multiple small, solid, homogeneous renal masses are consistent with nephroblastomatosis.
- *Wilms tumor:* Can be multiple and bilateral, but tends to be more heterogeneous.
- *Lymphoma/leukemia:* Can be bilateral, but tends to be infiltrative rather than discrete.

■ Essential Facts

- Multiple or diffuse nephrogenic rests within the kidneys can be a precursor to Wilms tumor.
- Rare after 7 years of age.
- Usually asymptomatic or presents as a flank mass.
- Can be seen in patients with certain syndromes, including hemihypertrophy, Beckwith-Wiedemann syndrome, trisomy 18, and sporadic aniridia.
- Most cases spontaneously regress, but in up to one-third of patients, Wilms tumor can develop.
- Ultrasound (US) screening every 3 months is typically performed until age 7 to detect the development of Wilms tumor.

- US: Hypoechoic or isoechoic to renal parenchyma.
- CT: Homogeneous and of low attenuation; enhances less than normal renal tissue.

■ Other Imaging Findings

- Multiple homogeneous masses can occur in the medulla or cortex of the kidney, but more frequently in the cortex. They can be as large as several centimeters.
- Also can appear as a subcapsular rind of soft tissue.
- Magnetic resonance imaging: T1—isointense to renal parenchyma; T2—isointense to slightly hyperintense to renal parenchyma; enhances less than normal renal parenchyma.

✓ Pearls & ✗ Pitfalls

- ✓ Nephroblastomatosis gives rise to one-third of Wilms tumors.
- ✓ It is found in nearly all bilateral Wilms tumors.
- ✗ It can be difficult to differentiate from Wilms tumor; however, Wilms tumor tends to be heterogeneous, whereas nephroblastomatosis is usually homogeneous.

Case 48

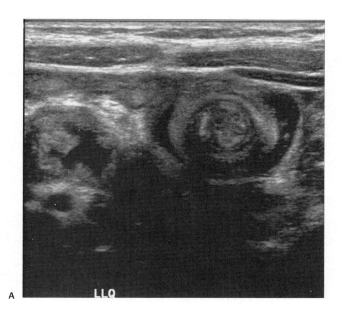

A

▪ Clinical Presentation

A toddler with episodic abdominal pain and "currant jelly" stools.

Further Work-up

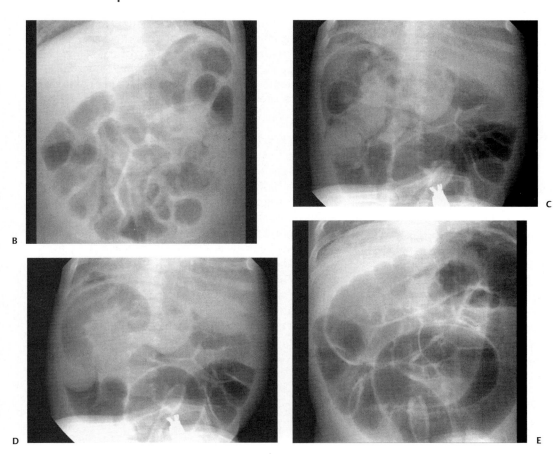

B

C

D

E

■ Imaging Findings

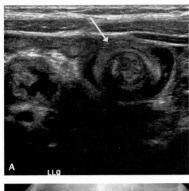
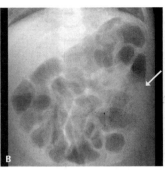
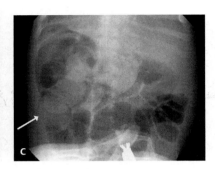
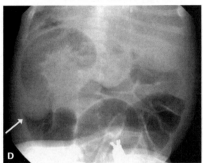
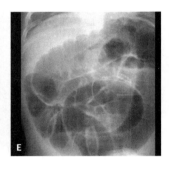

(A) A transverse sonographic image of the left lower quadrant demonstrates a mass with concentric rings of hyperechogenicity and hypoechogenicity, the so-called target sign (*arrow*). **(B–E)** Four fluoroscopic images obtained during an air reduction enema (with the patient in the prone position in C and D) demonstrate a sausage-like soft-tissue mass in the descending colon (*arrows*) that is progressively reduced proximally through the colon and end with disappearance of the soft-tissue mass and free reflux of air through the small bowel.

■ Differential Diagnosis

- **Intussusception:** The target sign is essentially diagnostic of intussusception, and in this case, the intussusception is not located in the right side of the abdomen because it has progressed distally into the descending colon.
- *Appendicitis:* May also be associated with a soft-tissue mass, but this is typically located in the right lower quadrant and does not demonstrate the target sign.
- *Meckel diverticulum:* May also cause intermittent abdominal pain and an abdominal mass, but it should not be associated with the target sign unless it has acted as a lead point in causing intussusception.

■ Essential Facts

- Intussusception is the most common abdominal emergency in infants and toddlers.
- Eighty percent of all cases present before the age of 2 years.
- It is rare before 3 months and after 6 years of age.
- Patients present with inconsolable crying, intermittent abdominal pain and vomiting, currant jelly stools (from mucosal hemorrhage), and a palpable mass.
- "Telescoping" of proximal bowel and accompanying mesentery into distal bowel, causing progressive lymphatic, venous, and eventually arterial insufficiency, can progress to necrosis, perforation, and peritonitis.
- Ninety percent of cases are ileocolic.
- Of these, 90% are idiopathic, likely related to lymphoid hypertrophy.
- Commonly identifiable lead points include Meckel diverticulum, appendicitis, lymphoma, and enteric duplications.
- In experienced hands, sonography is highly accurate.

■ Other Imaging Findings

- Plain radiographic findings are typically nonspecific, with a paucity of bowel gas in the right lower quadrant and possibly a soft-tissue mass and/or small-bowel obstruction.
- Computed tomography is not the examination of choice in suspected intussusception but shows a colonic mass with concentric rings of high and low attenuation.
- An enema may be performed with air or liquid contrast (not barium because of the possibility of perforation and barium peritonitis) and functions both diagnostically and therapeutically.

✓ Pearls & ✗ Pitfalls

- ✓ If intussusception is present, left lateral decubitus images will not show complete air filling of the ascending colon.
- ✓ Plain radiographs may show a "meniscus sign," with a soft-tissue mass bulging into the lumen of an air-containing colon.
- ✓ Enema reduction has 90% success rate, with a risk for perforation of less than 1%.
- ✓ Contraindications to attempted reduction include clinical findings of peritonitis or radiographic evidence of pneumoperitoneum.
- ✓ For pneumatic reduction, keep resting pressures below 120 mm Hg.
- ✓ Good rectal seal is crucial to prevent leakage of air or liquid contrast.

Case 49

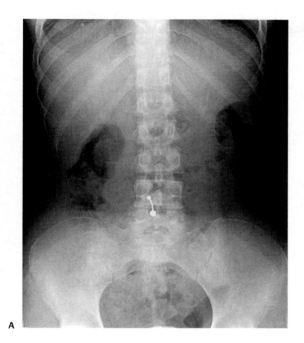

A

Clinical Presentation

A 13-year-old girl with right upper quadrant abdominal pain.

Further Work-up

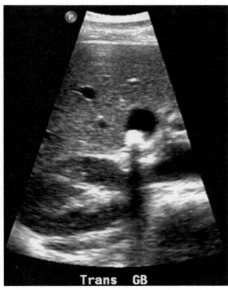

B Trans GB

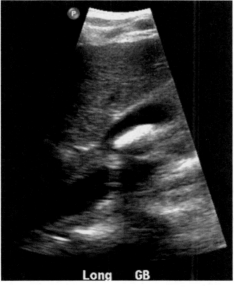

Long GB C

■ Imaging Findings

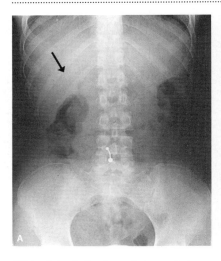 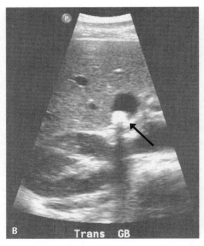 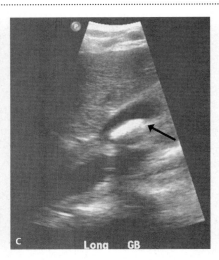

(A) An abdominal radiograph demonstrates a metallic belly button ring overlying the umbilicus. In the right upper quadrant are two round, calcific densities, likely representing gallstones (*arrow*). **(B,C)** Transverse and longitudinal sonograms of the right upper quadrant demonstrate round, echogenic, shadowing foci in the gallbladder lumen (*arrows*), consistent with gallstones. There is no gallbladder wall thickening, pericholecystic fluid, or other evidence of acute cholecystitis.

■ Differential Diagnosis

- **Cholelithiasis:** The finding of echogenic, shadowing foci in the gallbladder lumen, particularly if they move with changes in patient position, is diagnostic of cholelithiasis.
- *Biliary sludge:* Sludge may appear as layering echogenic material in the gallbladder lumen, but it usually does not appear as a round lesion and does not shadow; additionally, the degree of echogenicity is less than that of stones.
- *Gallbladder polyp:* Polyps may appear as discrete echogenic lesions, but they are uncommon in pediatric patients, are not as echogenic as stones, and do not move with changes in patient position.

■ Essential Facts

- Cholelithiasis is less common in children than in adults, but the incidence is increasing because of the rising prevalence of obesity (most common risk factor in pediatric patients).
- Persons at increased risk for cholesterol stones include Native Americans, women, patients on oral contraceptives, and patients on bowel rest or total parenteral nutrition.
- Pigment stones are less common, but risk factors include hemolytic anemias, infection of the biliary tree, and hypersplenism.
- At least 80% of patients with gallstones are asymptomatic.
- Patients present with postprandial right upper quadrant pain or symptoms of biliary obstruction.

■ Other Imaging Findings

- Fewer than 15% of gallstones are visible on plain radiographs.
- Sonography is extremely accurate in diagnosing cholelithiasis, with slightly lower accuracy in diagnosing choledocholithiasis and cholecystitis.
- Computed tomography and magnetic resonance imaging can also reliably detect stones and cholecystitis, although ultrasound is the first-line study to detect these lesions.
- Nuclear medicine is of value not to detect stones but to evaluate for cholecystitis.

✓ Pearls & ✗ Pitfalls

- ✓ To distinguish stones from polyps, verify mobility with change in patient position.
- ✗ Inspect the biliary duct to avoid missing choledocholithiasis.

Case 50

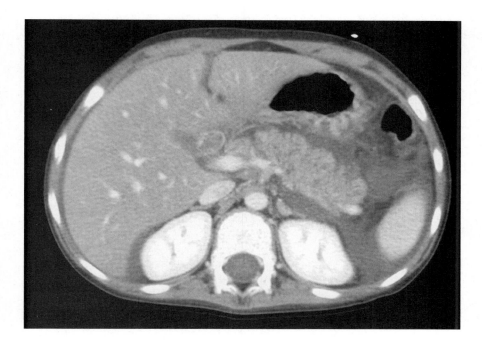

■ Clinical Presentation

Severe epigastric pain in a child on chemotherapy for acute lymphocytic leukemia.

■ Imaging Findings

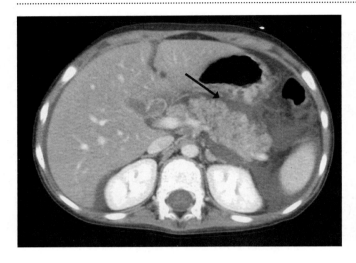

An axial post-contrast computed tomography (CT) image of the upper abdomen demonstrates a swollen, heterogeneous, edematous-appearing pancreas (*arrow*) with surrounding fluid and inflammatory changes and a small amount of ascites. Neither the pancreatic nor the biliary ducts are dilated.

■ Differential Diagnosis

- *Acute pancreatitis:* The inflammatory changes in the pancreas are diagnostic of pancreatitis, and the lack of ductal dilatation argues against an obstructive etiology.
- *Traumatic pancreatitis:* Patients who have been subjected to abuse may present with pancreatitis secondary to epigastric trauma, and it is important to consider this possibility in infants and small children with no other predisposing conditions.
- *Anomalies of the pancreatic ductal system:* Annular pancreas, certain types of choledochal cyst, and other anatomic anomalies may present with acute pancreatitis and should be suspected in cases with no known predisposing conditions.

■ Essential Facts

- The incidence is lower in children than adults, in part because the two main causes in adults—alcohol abuse and gallstones—are less prevalent in children.
- Causes include trauma, anatomic anomalies, infection, medications (as in this case), and hereditary disorders such as cystic fibrosis.
- Patients present with abdominal pain, vomiting, tenderness, and acute abdomen.
- The most common complication is pseudocyst.
- CT is preferable to evaluate the extent of disease.

■ Other Imaging Findings

- Sonography is the first-line study.
- Magnetic resonance cholangiopancreatography offers superb visualization of the pancreatic and biliary ductal systems.

✓ Pearls & ✗ Pitfalls

- ✓ Pancreatitis is associated with elevated serum levels of amylase and lipase (the latter is more specific).
- ✓ The diagnosis is clinical, but imaging is often performed to rule out other pathologies, assess for predisposing conditions (e.g., gallstones), rule out complications (e.g., pseudocysts), and provide prognostic assessment.

Case 51

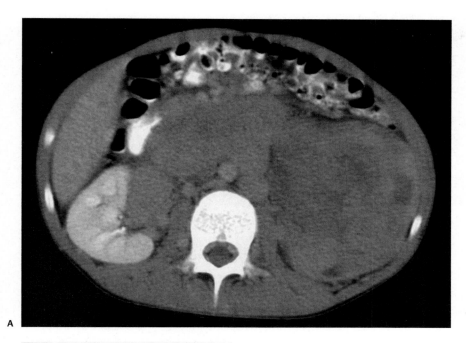

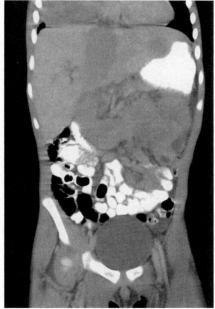

▓ Clinical Presentation

A 3-year-old child with a palpable left-sided abdominal mass.

■ Imaging Findings

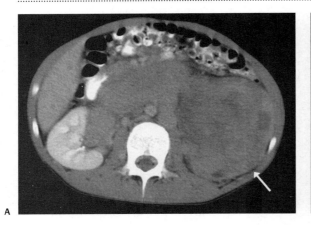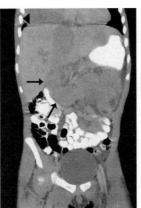

(A,B) Axial and coronal reformat images of a computed tomography (CT) abdominal examination demonstrate a large, heterogeneous mass in the left renal fossa, with abnormal dilatation and a continuous filling defect in the left renal vein, inferior vena cava (IVC), and inferior part of the right atrium (*black and white arrows*). In addition, there is a large soft-tissue mass in the base of the right hemithorax (*arrowhead*).

■ Differential Diagnosis

- **Wilms tumor:** A large, heterogeneous renal mass replacing much of the kidney is typical of Wilms tumor, which in this case has invaded the left renal vein and extended up the IVC into the right atrium. In addition, there is a large right lower lobe pulmonary metastasis.
- *Neuroblastoma:* This lesion can also present as a large heterogeneous mass in the renal fossa, but it usually displaces the kidney inferiorly, is considerably more likely to show calcifications, and does not invade the renal vein or metastasize to the lungs.
- *Mesoblastic nephroma:* This solid mass, which can appear identical to Wilms tumor, is found in neonates.

■ Essential Facts

- Wilms tumor is the most common renal malignancy and solid abdominal malignancy of childhood.
- The median age of patients is 3 years.
- The tumor usually presents as a large abdominal mass.
- Ten percent of cases are bilateral.
- Wilms tumor tends to metastasize to the lungs.
- CT is an excellent assessment tool and is usually indicated for the staging of chest disease.

■ Other Imaging Findings

- Sonography is the first-line imaging modality in young patients with an abdominal mass and provides an excellent assessment for vascular invasion.
- Magnetic resonance imaging is also excellent.

✓ Pearls & ✗ Pitfalls

- ✓ The tumor arises from persistent metanephric blastema.
- ✓ In contrast to neuroblastoma, Wilms tumor rarely causes skeletal metastases.
- ✓ Chemotherapy often used to shrink the tumor before resection.
- ✓ The current cure rate in the United States is better than 90%.

Case 52

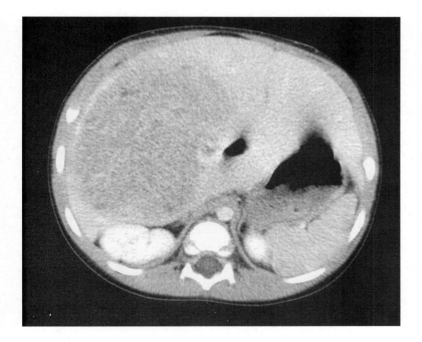

▣ Clinical Presentation

A 1-year-old with a right-sided abdominal mass.

■ Imaging Findings

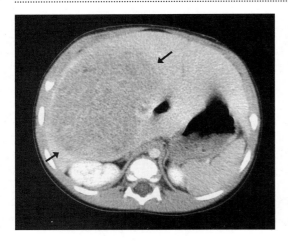

Axial computed tomography image obtained after the intravenous administration of contrast demonstrates a large, heterogeneous, hypoattenuating mass occupying most of the liver (*arrows*).

■ Differential Diagnosis

- **Hepatoblastoma:** This lesion tends to present as a large, clearly circumscribed, hypodense liver mass, often with calcifications (although they are not seen in this case).
- *Metastasis:* Several pediatric malignancies can present with a large hepatic metastasis, although the lesions tend to be multiple and the primary tumor is usually apparent on other images. Common culprits include neuroblastoma and Wilms tumor.
- *Hepatocellular carcinoma:* This lesion can have an identical appearance but rarely occurs in patients this young. It becomes the most common primary liver malignancy after the age of 4 years.

■ Essential Facts

- Most hepatoblastomas are quite large at presentation.
- Perhaps because they arise from embryonic cells, most lesions present before 18 months of age.
- Hepatoblastoma is associated with elevated levels of the tumor marker α-fetoprotein.

■ Other Imaging Findings

- Ultrasound demonstrates a large, well-defined, hypervascular, hypoechoic mass.
- On magnetic resonance imaging, there is a low signal on T1 and a high signal on T2, with heterogeneous contrast enhancement.

✓ Pearls & ✗ Pitfalls

- ✓ Imaging features alone are not specific but help to define the extent for surgical planning and to assess the treatment response.

Case 53

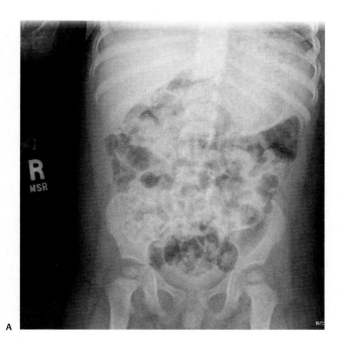

A

■ Clinical Presentation

A young girl with abdominal pain and an epigastric mass.

Further Work-up

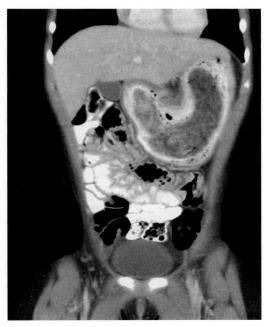

B

■ **Imaging Findings**

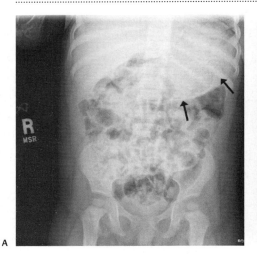 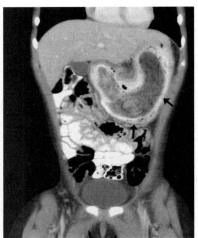

A   B

(A) Abdominal radiograph demonstrates a heterogeneous soft-tissue mass in the shape of the stomach (*arrows*). **(B)** Coronal reformat computed tomography image of the abdomen after oral and intravenous administration of contrast demonstrates a large, heterogeneous, hypodense gastric filling defect (*arrow*) that conforms to the shape of the stomach and is surrounded by oral contrast material, indicating that it does not arise from the gastric wall. It contains hypodense pockets of gas.

■ **Differential Diagnosis**

- *Bezoar:* The gastric shape, heterogeneity, and lack of connection of the lesion to the gastric wall are essentially diagnostic of a bezoar. This patient's bezoar was composed of hair.
- *Postprandial state:* A patient who consumes a large meal just before imaging may also demonstrate a large stomach containing heterogeneous material, although this should not persist over time.
- *Gastroparesis:* Patients with impaired gastric emptying may demonstrate similar findings for a prolonged period.

■ **Essential Facts**

- Bezoars are due to the retention and accumulation of ingested material in the gastric lumen.
- They are associated with impaired gastric emptying.
- Types include phytobezoar (plant material; for example, persimmon), lactobezoar (milk or formula), and trichobezoar (hair).

✓ **Pearls & ✗ Pitfalls**

✓ Patients with trichobezoars may have hair loss.
✓ Trichobezoars are more common in girls, particularly in the setting of psychiatric conditions.
✓ Hair extending from the stomach into the duodenum is known as *Rapunzel syndrome.*
✓ In some cultures, animal bezoars were considered precious and used to treat diseases.
✓ Bezoars can be complicated by ulceration, hemorrhage, and perforation.

Case 54

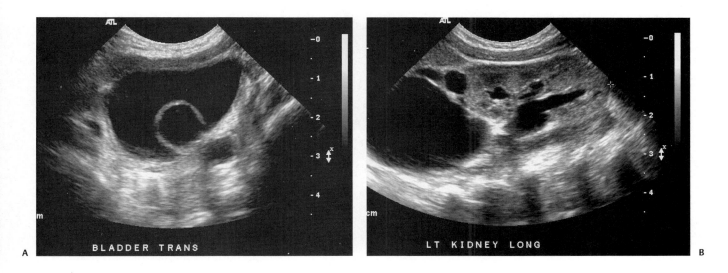

A BLADDER TRANS

B LT KIDNEY LONG

■ Clinical Presentation

An infant with a recent history of urinary tract infection.

Further Work-up

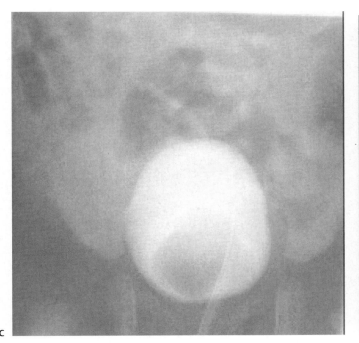

C

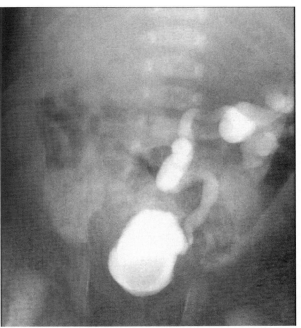

D

■ Imaging Findings

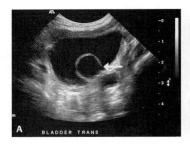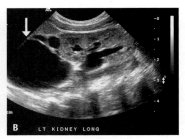

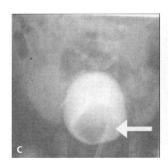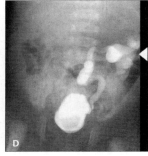

(A,B) A transverse sonogram through the urinary bladder demonstrates a cystic structure adjacent to the expected location of the left ureterovesical junction (*arrow*), almost certainly representing a ureterocele, and a longitudinal sonogram of the left kidney demonstrates mild lower pole hydronephrosis and severe upper pole hydronephrosis (*arrow*). **(C,D)** Two radiographic images from a voiding cysto-urethrogram demonstrate a filling defect in the bladder, corresponding to the ureterocele seen on sonography (*arrow*), as well as a grade 4 reflect into the lower pole of the left kidney (*arrowhead*), which is inferiorly displaced by the hydronephrotic (obstructed) upper pole.

■ Differential Diagnosis

- **Complete ureteral duplication with upper pole ureterocele:** The filling defect in the bladder has a typical appearance of a ureterocele, and the difference in the degrees of hydronephrosis between the upper and lower poles establishes the diagnosis of duplication with obstruction of drainage from the upper pole by the ureterocele. The inferior displacement of the lower pole collecting system by the obstructed upper pole is the "drooping lilly" sign.
- *Bladder mass:* Hematomas, fungus balls, and rhabdomyosarcomas can present as bladder filling defects, but they should not be anechoic centrally and are not associated with ureteral duplication.
- *Extrinsic impression on the bladder:* Bowel indenting the bladder can sometimes mimic a filling defect, although an oblique or lateral image will quickly prove that the apparent mass is not intraluminal.

■ Essential Facts

- Ureteroceles are five times more common in girls than boys and bilateral in 10% of patients.
- Ureteral duplication is two times more common in girls, and complete duplications are bilateral in 40%.
- Upper pole hydronephrosis has either of two possible causes: an obstructing ureterocele or ectopic insertion into such sites as the urethra, vagina, and vas deferens.

✓ Pearls & ✗ Pitfalls

- ✓ A duplex system, as opposed to a duplication, is one in which two pelvocalyceal systems drain into a single ureter.
- ✓ In complete ureteral duplication, the Meyer-Weigert rule states that the ectopic upper pole ureter inserts inferomedially to the lower pole ureter.
- ✓ The more ectopic the ureteral insertion, the more dysplastic the upper pole of the kidney.
- ✓ Ectopic ureters cause incontinence in girls when they insert below the sphincter, and such female patients may present with around-the-clock wetting.

Case 55

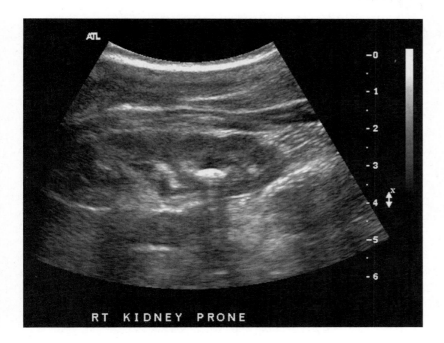

Clinical Presentation

A child with right flank pain and hematuria.

■ Imaging Findings

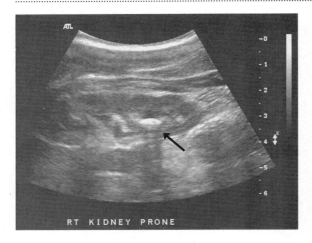

RT KIDNEY PRONE

A longitudinal sonogram of the right kidney demonstrates an echogenic focus in the inferior portion of the collecting system with acoustic shadowing (*arrow*). There is no evidence of urinary obstruction.

■ Differential Diagnosis

- *Nephrolithiasis:* Kidney stones, like stones elsewhere in the body, typically appear echogenic and cast acoustic shadows on sonography.
- *Blood clot:* Hematomas may appear hyperechoic, but they generally do not cast acoustic shadows. They are typically associated with bleeding diatheses, recent trauma or surgery, or tumors or stones.
- *Fungus ball:* These lesions also appear echogenic and may shadow, but they are generally found in immunocompromised patients.

■ Essential Facts

- Stones are less common in children than adults, although they are being recognized more frequently than in the past.
- In children, causes such as urinary tract anomalies (e.g., ureteropelvic junction obstruction), inborn errors of metabolism (e.g., cystinuria), infection, and inflammatory bowel disease are relatively more common than in adults.
- The classic presentation of acute renal colic is less common in children, particularly young children, although most do present with abdominal pain.
- The most common types of stones in pediatric patients include calcium oxalate (50%), calcium phosphate (25%), and struvite (magnesium ammonium phosphate, 10%).
- Struvite stones are associated with infection by urease-producing organisms such as *Proteus*.
- Ultrasound is excellent for demonstrating stones in the kidney and urinary bladder and should generally be the first-line imaging modality in children, although nonobstructive stones in the ureter may be difficult to detect.

■ Other Imaging Findings

- Noncontrast computed tomography is the most sensitive technique.
- Intravenous urography should no longer play a role in the evaluation of pediatric nephrolithiasis, except in very unusual circumstances.

✓ Pearls & ✗ Pitfalls

- ✓ The two most common sites where stones become lodged are the ureteropelvic junction and the ureterovesical junction.
- ✓ The finding of stones in a pediatric patient without known risk factors such as obstruction or infection should generally prompt a metabolic work-up.

Case 56

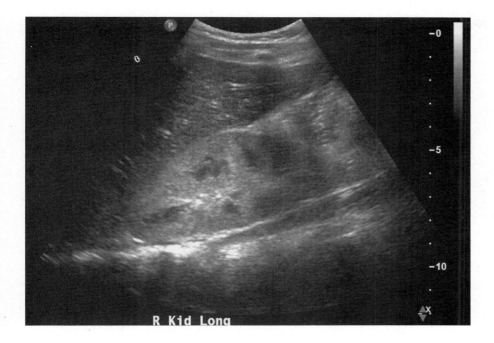

R Kid Long

■ Clinical Presentation

A young child with a history of bloody diarrhea, disseminated intravascular coagulation, and acute renal failure.

■ Imaging Findings

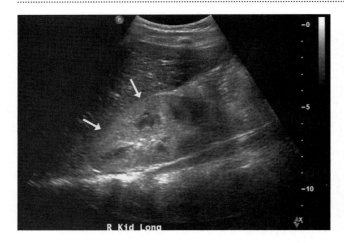

A longitudinal sonogram of the right kidney demonstrates hyperechogenicity of the upper and middle portions of the right kidney (*arrows*), without evidence of obstruction. The left kidney (not shown) also demonstrated areas of increased echogenicity.

■ Differential Diagnosis

- ***Hemolytic-uremic syndrome:*** The renal imaging findings are nonspecific but typical of infection or vasculitis. The associated findings of bloody diarrhea and acute renal failure are strongly suggestive of hemolytic-uremic syndrome.
- *Pyelonephritis:* Multifocal bilateral pyelonephritis, more likely due to bacteremia than to vesico-ureteral reflux, could produce a similar imaging appearance.
- *Henoch-Schönlein purpura:* This multisystem vasculitis can be accompanied by similar renal manifestations, although it is more often associated with purpuric rash, gastrointestinal problems (including intussusception), and arthritis.

■ Essential Facts

- The peak incidence is at 6 months to 4 years of age.
- Most patients present with acute bloody diarrhea and a low urine output.
- The syndrome is related to infection by enterohemorrhagic *Escherichia coli* O157.
- At least 85% of patients recover with supportive care.

✓ Pearls & ✗ Pitfalls

- ✓ This is not an imaging diagnosis, although imaging may be ordered to rule out urinary tract obstruction as a possible cause of oliguria.
- ✓ Renal calcification may be a sequela.

Case 57

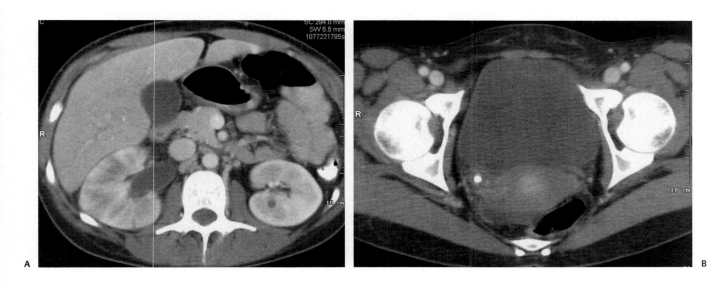

A

B

■ Clinical Presentation

A teenager with high fever and flank pain.

■ Imaging Findings

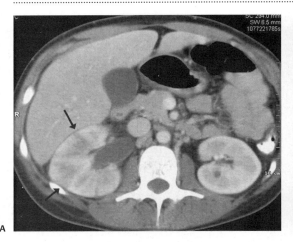 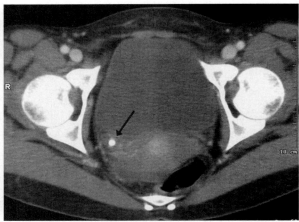

(A,B) Axial computed tomography images at the level of the kidneys and urinary bladder after oral and intravenous contrast demonstrate a swollen right kidney with wedge-shaped areas of parenchymal hypoattenuation ("striated nephrogram," *arrow*) and hydronephrosis. In addition, a several-millimeter calcific density is seen at the right ureterovesical junction (UVJ, *arrow*).

■ Differential Diagnosis

- **Obstructive uropathy:** In the clinical setting of high-grade fever and flank pain, the striated nephrogram is essentially diagnostic of pyelonephritis, and the hydronephrosis and UVJ stone establish that the infection is related to obstruction.
- *Renal infarction:* Acute embolic renal infarction can produce swelling and areas of hypoattenuation but should not be associated with fever and stone.
- *Nephroblastomatosis:* This condition, associated with Wilms tumor, can present with multiple areas of hypoattenuation within the renal parenchyma but should not be associated with fever or stones.

■ Essential Facts

- This is an acute infection of the renal parenchyma.
- It is more common in girls than in boys.
- Routes by which bacteria can reach the kidneys include vesicoureteral reflux (*Escherichia coli*), hematogenous dissemination (*Staphylococcus aureus*), and direct inoculation.
- The most common causative organism is *E. coli.*
- Complications include abscess, sepsis, and renal scarring, which may be followed by hypertension and renal insufficiency later in life.

✓ Pearls & ✗ Pitfalls

- ✓ An infected, obstructed kidney is a urologic emergency that is usually treated by image-guided percutaneous nephrostomy.
- ✓ Patients with pyelonephritis should be assessed with renal sonography and voiding cysto-urethrography.
- ✓ Nuclear medicine renal scintigraphy is more sensitive than sonography for the detection of scarring.

Case 58

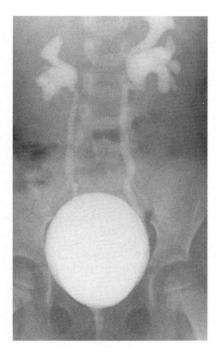

■ Clinical Presentation

A child with a recent history of urinary tract infection.

■ Imaging Findings

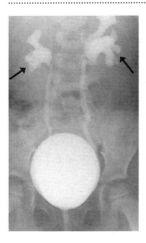

A radiograph from a voiding cystourethrogram (VCUG) demonstrates bilateral vesicoureteral reflux during voiding (*arrows*).

■ Differential Diagnosis

- **Vesicoureteral reflux:** Assuming that an initial scout radiograph of the abdomen demonstrated no contrast material in the abdomen, these findings are diagnostic of vesicoureteral reflux. This degree of calyceal blunting and ureteral dilatation is consistent with grade 3 reflux.
- *Normal bowel or bone anatomy:* Depending on the distribution of bowel gas and the degree of obliquity of the images, normal anatomy can sometimes mimic a contrast-opacified ureter, although that would not be a reasonable hypothesis in this case.
- *Prior administration of contrast:* Inexperienced observers sometimes mistakenly interpret the radiographic findings of patients who have received intravenous contrast material as vesicoureteral reflux. In general, there will be opacification of the renal parenchyma in such cases, and it would be rare for both ureters to be as well opacified as in this case.

■ Essential Facts

- During VCUG, iodinated contrast material is infused retrograde into the urinary bladder via a urethral catheter.
- Vesicoureteral reflux can cause bacteria to spread from the urinary bladder into the ureter and kidney.
- Most cases of vesicoureteral reflux result from an abnormally short, angulated segment of a ureter within the bladder wall.
- Vesicoureteral reflux is estimated to be present in up to 2% of the pediatric population, although the percentage is higher in patients with a history of pyelonephritis.
- Vesicoureteral reflux is more common in girls than in boys, and less common in blacks than in whites.
- Classification:
  - Grade 1: reflux into the ureter that does not ascend to the renal pelvis
  - Grade 2: reflux into a nondilated renal collecting system
  - Grade 3: mild blunting of the renal calyces
  - Grade 4: further increased dilatation of the collecting system and ureter
  - Grade 5: further increased dilatation with intrarenal reflux
- Most cases of vesicoureteral reflux resolve spontaneously over several years, although this is less likely in patients with higher grades of reflux and in older patients. Therefore, the prevalence of reflux is inversely proportional to age.
- Long-term sequelae can include renal insufficiency and hypertension, which are most likely in patients with severe or long-term reflux associated with urinary tract infections.
- Treatments include the prophylactic daily administration of antibiotics until the child outgrows the reflux, endoscopic injection of material to increase the competency of the ureterovesical junction, and surgical reimplantation of the ureter.

✓ Pearls & ✗ Pitfalls

- ✓ Obtain an early filling view of the bladder to avoid missing filling defects that can become obscured as the bladder continues to fill.
- ✓ Vesicoureteral reflux can be diagnosed by sonography when transient or variable hydronephrosis is observed during the course of the examination.
- ✓ The incidence of vesico-reteral reflux is higher (~30%) in the siblings of patients with reflux than in the general population.
- ✓ Vesicoureteral reflux is more common in children with neurogenic bladders and voiding dysfunction.
- ✗ Avoid catheters with balloons because they can be mistaken for intraluminal filling defects such as a ureterocele.

Case 59

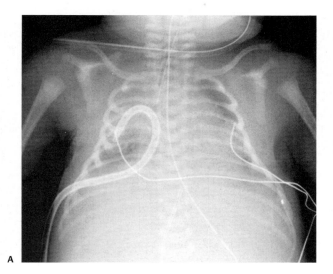

A

■ Clinical Presentation

A newborn with a prenatal history of oligohydramnios presenting with bilateral pneumothoraces and bilateral abdominal masses.

Further Work-up

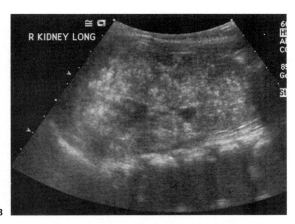

B

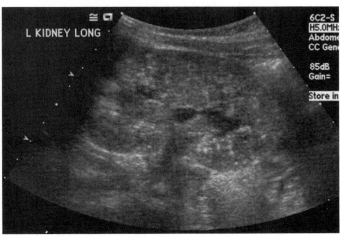

C

◼ Imaging Findings

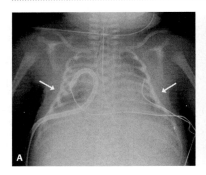 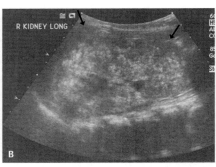 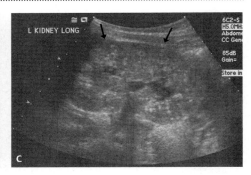

(A) A frontal chest radiograph demonstrates a bell-shaped thorax, consistent with pulmonary hypoplasia (*arrows*). **(B,C)** Bilateral longitudinal renal sonograms demonstrate markedly enlarged kidneys with poor corticomedullary differentiation and a relatively hypoechoic peripheral renal cortex compared with the rest of the renal parenchyma (*arrows*).

◼ Differential Diagnosis

- ***Autosomal-recessive polycystic kidney disease:*** Patients with this disorder frequently have a history of oligohydramnios and hypoplastic lungs (because of decreased fetal urine production), and the sonographic findings are characteristic.
- *Autosomal-dominant polycystic disease:* Patients with this disorder usually present much later in life, with no history of significant impairment of renal function as children, normal parenchymal echogenicity, and discrete cysts.
- *Cystic renal dysplasia:* This can cause poor corticomedullary differentiation, but the lesion is associated with long-standing obstruction or infection, and the kidneys should be smaller than normal.

◼ Essential Facts

- Although the term *polycystic* is used, the cysts are generally too small to be seen by radiologic studies.
- The condition is related to ectasia of the distal nephrons, associated with flattening of the epithelium.
- It typically presents early in life, but milder forms exist that present in childhood and adolescence.
- Eighty percent of infants who survive longer than 1 month will live at least 15 years.
- Autosomal-recessive polycystic kidney disease is related to a defective fibrocystin gene on chromosome 6.
- It is associated with congenital hepatic fibrosis, which eventually causes portal hypertension.
- Enlarged kidneys and oligohydramnios are frequently detected on prenatal sonography.

✓ Pearls & ✗ Pitfalls

- ✓ Both kidneys should be symmetrically involved.
- ✓ Long-term survival requires both liver and kidney transplants.

Case 60

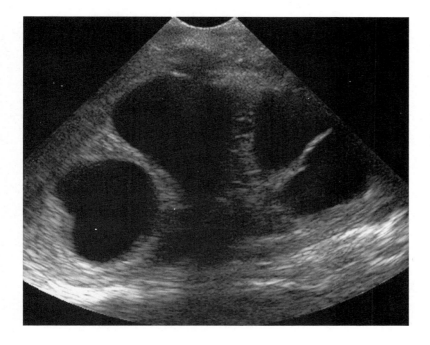

■ Clinical Presentation

A 10-year-old with a flank mass.

■ Imaging Findings

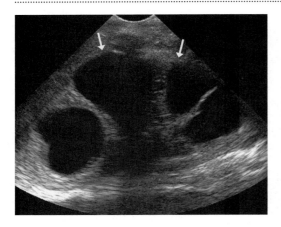

A longitudinal sonogram of the right kidney demonstrates multiple large renal cysts that do not connect with one another or the renal pelvis (*arrows*). The left kidney had a virtually identical appearance.

■ Differential Diagnosis

- **Autosomal-dominant polycystic disease:** The finding of multiple large renal cysts bilaterally is typical of this disorder.
- *Simple renal cysts:* These lesions are much less frequent in children than in older adults and should not be as numerous or as large as the ones in this case. In addition, renal function should be completely normal.
- *Tuberous sclerosis:* Multiple renal cysts are often present, but these are typically associated with renal angiomyolipomata, and the patient should manifest other stigmata of the disorder, such as skin lesions, seizures, and mental retardation.

■ Essential Facts

- This disorder is at least 20 times more common than autosomal-recessive polycystic disease and occurs in 1 in 500 births.
- Approximately 10% of cases are the consequence of spontaneous mutations.
- The mean age at diagnosis is approximately 40 years.
- Autosomal-dominant polycystic disease is a major cause of chronic renal failure in older adults.
- Approximately half of patients have detectable cysts in the first 10 years of life.
- The condition is related to cystic dilatation of the proximal nephrons.
- The cysts communicate with nephrons and contain urine.
- Cysts are often found in other organs, such as the liver and pancreas.

✓ Pearls & ✗ Pitfalls

- ✓ The condition is associated with cerebrovascular anomalies such as berry aneurysms.
- ✓ Patients may present with pain because of cystic hemorrhage or infection.

Case 61

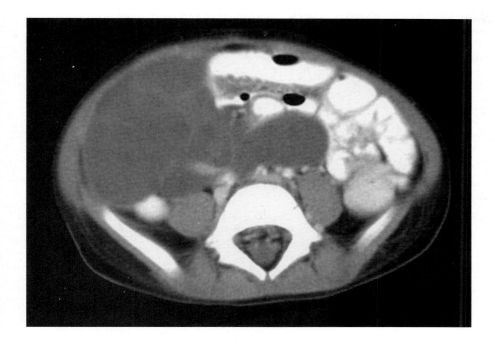

■ Clinical Presentation

A child with a large, soft, right-sided abdominal mass.

■ Imaging Findings

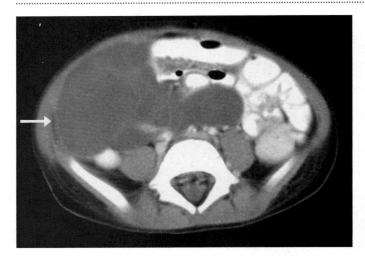

Post-contrast abdominal computed tomography (CT) image demonstrates a large, well-circumscribed, predominately fluid-density, multiseptate abdominal mass (*arrow*) displacing viscera to the left.

■ Differential Diagnosis

- *Lymphatic malformation:* The CT appearance in this case is typical of a lymph-containing, multicystic lesion.
- *Abscess:* Abscesses can have a multiseptate appearance, but the patient has no clinical signs of infection, the septa are very thin and do not enhance well, and there is no surrounding inflammation.
- *Venous malformation:* These lesions may appear to be of fluid density and multiseptate on a single CT image, but multiple images generally demonstrate more enhancement and multiple tubular structures within them.

■ Essential Facts

- Lymphatic malformations account for 25% of all benign vascular tumors of childhood.
- They are commonly called *cystic hygromas* when they involve the head and neck (75%).
- The lesions consist of obstructed lymphatic channels, which may grow progressively more distended with time.
- They are associated with numerous conditions, including Turner syndrome, Down syndrome, and Noonan syndrome.
- They are rarely life-threatening and are often treated for cosmetic reasons.
- Lymphatic malformations can be surgically excised or treated with a sclerosant percutaneously.

■ Other Imaging Findings

- Sonography demonstrates no internal flow.
- Magnetic resonance imaging is best for determining the extent of a lesion; there is no contrast enhancement, although the fluid intensity may vary depending on hemorrhage.

✓ Pearls & ✗ Pitfalls

- ✓ May enlarge suddenly or become painful because of hemorrhage
- ✓ Will recur if merely drained

Case 62

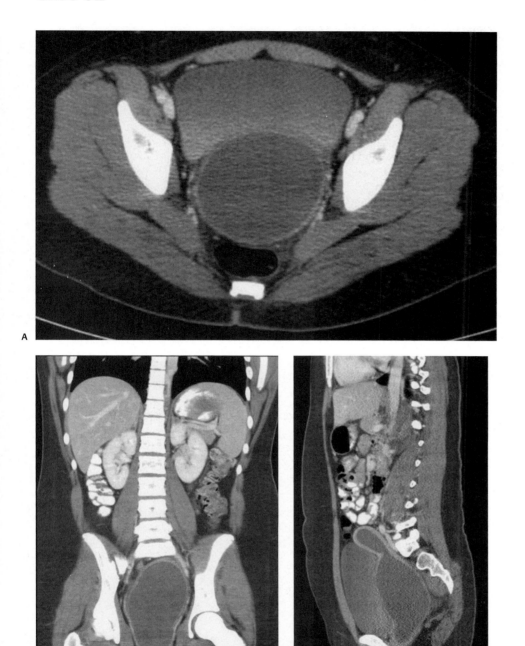

A

B

C

■ Clinical Presentation

A teenage girl with primary amenorrhea and a pelvic mass.

Imaging Findings

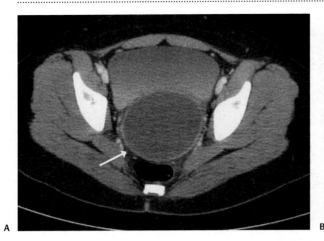
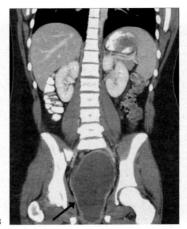
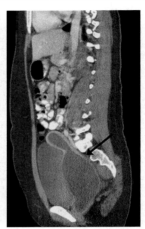

(A–C) Sagittal, axial, and coronal post-contrast computed tomography images demonstrate a large, fluid-filled mass with enhancing walls in the expected location of the vagina and uterus (*arrows*).

Differential Diagnosis

- **Hydrometrocolpos:** The location of the lesion between the urinary bladder and rectum, the inability to identify the vagina and uterus separate from the lesion, and the presence of fluid within the enhancing, thin-walled, caudally positioned vagina and more thick-walled, cranially positioned uterus are typical.
- *Abscess:* A pelvic abscess in the rectovesical space resulting from a process such as perforated appendicitis or pelvic inflammatory disease could have a similar appearance, but here the clinical presentation is inconsistent and there is no evidence of surrounding inflammation.
- *Cystic ovarian tumor:* These lesions can present as cystic pelvic masses in patients with no evidence of infection, but the uterus should be easily identified separate from the lesion.

Essential Facts

- Hydrometrocolpos results from menstruation into an obstructed vagina or uterus.
- Vaginal obstruction may be secondary to imperforate hymen, vaginal atresia, or cervical stenosis.
- Mass effect can cause bladder outlet obstruction.
- Hydrometrocolpos may also present in the neonatal period as a pelvic mass because of maternal hormonal stimulation.

Other Imaging Findings

- Sonography may show a fluid-fluid level in the distended vagina or uterus.
- Magnetic resonance imaging is useful to assess for urogenital tract anomalies, such as septate or bicornuate uterus and renal agenesis.

✓ Pearls & ✗ Pitfalls

- ✓ It is important to distinguish clinically between a history of primary amenorrhea (absence of menstruation by the age of 16 years in a girl who has otherwise grown and developed normally) and secondary amenorrhea (cessation of menstrual periods for at least 6 months in a patient who is not pregnant, breastfeeding, or in menopause).

Case 63

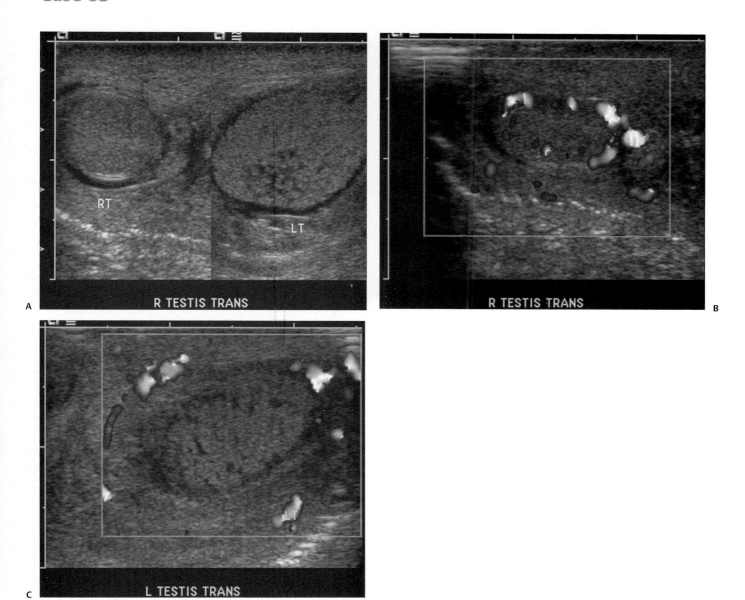

A

R TESTIS TRANS

B

R TESTIS TRANS

C

L TESTIS TRANS

■ Clinical Presentation

A 12-year-old boy with acute scrotal pain and vomiting.

■ Imaging Findings

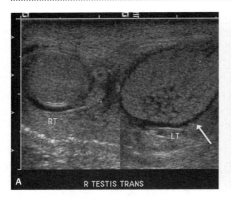 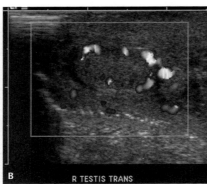 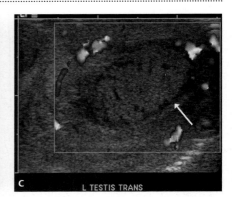

(A–C) Transverse gray-scale and Doppler images of both testes demonstrate an enlarged, heterogeneously hypoechoic left testis with no internal blood flow (*arrows*).

■ Differential Diagnosis

- **Testicular torsion:** The combination of an enlarged, heterogeneously hypoechoic testis and no demonstrable internal color Doppler signal is essentially diagnostic of testicular torsion.
- *Epididymo-orchitis:* Inflammation of the testis can cause it to be enlarged and hypoechoic with increased surrounding blood flow, but in this condition the testis itself should also demonstrate normal to increased Doppler signal.
- *Torsion of the epididymal appendage:* This condition may also present with acute scrotal pain, but the testis itself demonstrates normal to increased blood flow, and it is usually possible to demonstrate a swollen, hypovascular epididymal appendage.

■ Essential Facts

- Testicular torsion is most common in infants and teenagers.
- It presents with acute pain and swelling.
- It is due to inadequate testicular fixation, which results from failure of the tunica vaginalis and testis to connect ("bell clapper deformity"), so that the testis can rotate around its vascular pedicle.
- Doppler sonography is the imaging examination of choice for scrotal pathology.
- Treatment is surgical, with detorsion and orchiopexy of a salvageable testis.

✓ Pearls & ✗ Pitfalls

- ✓ In patients with acute scrotal pain, epididymo-orchitis and torsion of the epididymal appendage are both more common than testicular torsion.
- ✓ Early diagnosis of torsion (within 6 hours) is important to salvage the testis.
- ✓ If torsion occurs, bell clapper deformity is typically bilateral, so orchiopexy is indicated for the contralateral testis.

Case 64

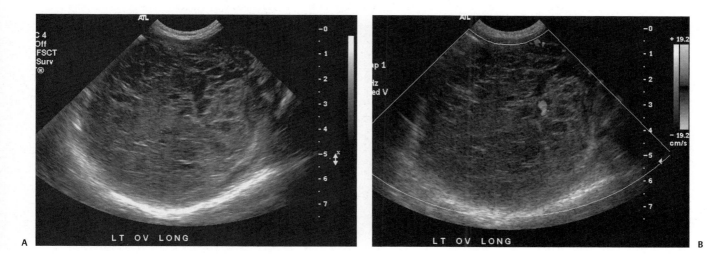

A

B

■ Clinical Presentation

A neonatal girl with an abdominal mass.

■ Imaging Findings

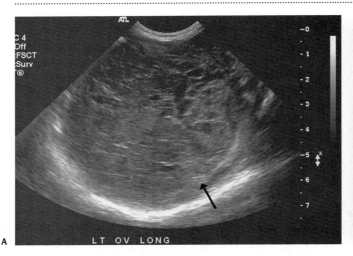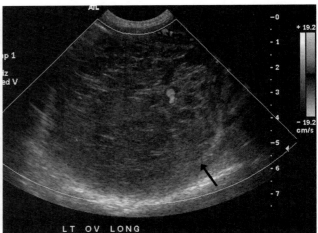

(A,B) Longitudinal gray-scale and Doppler sonograms of the pelvis demonstrate a markedly enlarged (> 6 cm in diameter), heterogeneously hypoechoic left ovary containing multiple peripheral cysts (*arrows*). The ovary shows almost no internal Doppler signal.

■ Differential Diagnosis

- **Ovarian torsion:** The finding of an enlarged ovary containing multiple cysts is typical of ovarian torsion.
- *Hemorrhagic ovarian cyst:* Ovarian cysts that hemorrhage may also present as pelvic masses, although it is usually possible to identify normal ovarian tissue adjacent to the cystic mass. Such cysts may be complicated by torsion.
- *Ovarian neoplasm:* This is not common in neonates and is generally associated with normal to increased blood flow.

■ Essential Facts

- Ovarian torsion is most common in pre- and peripubertal patients.
- Neonatal cases are due to maternal hormone stimulation and a relatively large size of the ovaries at birth.
- The presence of multiple cysts is related to venous congestion.
- Torsion is more likely in the presence of an ovarian mass.
- The treatment is surgical detorsion.

✓ Pearls & ✗ Pitfalls

- ✓ Sonography is the preferred imaging modality.
- ✓ Color Doppler evaluation is of limited utility, perhaps because the ovary has a dual blood supply, permitting some flow even in torsion.
- ✓ Cysts are often peripherally located.

Case 65

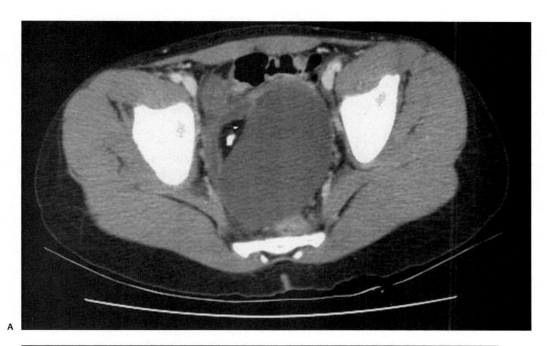

A

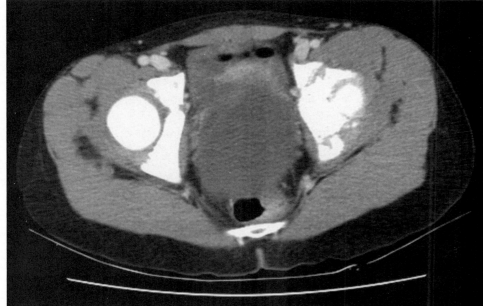

B

■ Clinical Presentation

An adolescent girl with right lower quadrant pain.

■ Imaging Findings

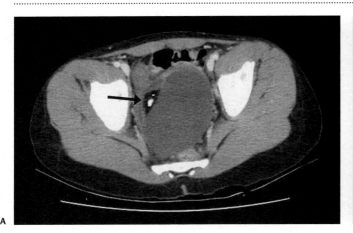
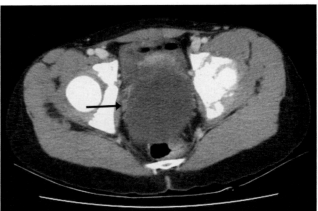

A   B

(A,B) Axial post-contrast computed tomography images demonstrate a cystic mass in the rectovesical space that has three different attenuation levels: calcium, fluid, and fat (*arrows*).

■ Differential Diagnosis

- ***Ovarian teratoma:*** The finding of an ovarian mass that contains calcium, fluid, and particularly fat is diagnostic of an ovarian teratoma.
- *Appendicitis:* An appendicolith can be mistaken for calcification in a teratoma, but the patient should have signs and symptoms of infection, and fat should not be present within the lesion itself.
- *Other ovarian neoplasm:* Other germ cell and epithelial carcinomas can present as ovarian masses, but these rarely contain calcification and almost never contain tissue with fat attenuation.

■ Essential Facts

- The name is derived from the Greek *terato-* ("monster") and *-oma* ("mass").
- This is the most common ovarian germ cell tumor.
- It contains ectodermal, mesodermal, and endodermal elements and may include formed hair and teeth.
- Most are benign.

■ Other Imaging Findings

- Plain radiographs may show calcifications or teeth in association with a pelvic mass.
- Sonography usually shows a heterogeneous mass that may contain a fluid-fluid level and calcifications.
- Magnetic resonance imaging can establish fat density within the lesion.

✓ Pearls & ✕ Pitfalls

- ✓ Ten percent are bilateral.
- ✓ Rupture can result in chemical peritonitis.

Case 66

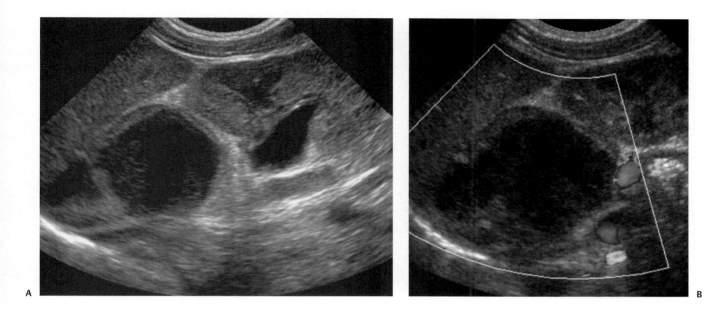

A   B

■ Clinical Presentation

A newborn with prenatal hydronephrosis.

■ Imaging Findings

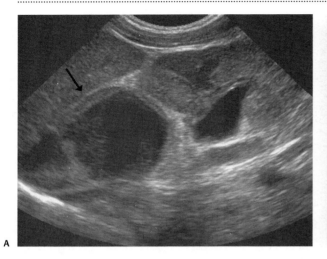
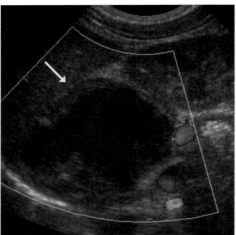

A   B

(A) Longitudinal gray-scale ultrasound (US) image: superior to the normal-appearing kidney is a large, predominately hypoechoic mass with a peripheral hyperechoic rim and internal debris (*arrow*). **(B)** Doppler US image: there is no blood flow within the lesion (*arrow*).

■ Differential Diagnosis

- ***Adrenal hemorrhage:*** An avascular mass in the adrenal bed with a mixed echotexture is consistent with hemorrhage.
- *Neuroblastoma:* Doppler US should show internal blood flow.
- *Congenital adrenal hyperplasia:* This should be a bilateral finding, and the normal contour of the adrenal gland is usually preserved.

■ Essential Facts

- Adrenal hemorrhage most often occurs in full-term and large-for-gestational age infants with a history of perinatal stress, such as birth trauma, asphyxia, sepsis, or coagulopathy.
- Patients may present with anemia, a drop in hematocrit, jaundice, or adrenal insufficiency.
- The usual treatment is observation only.
- Adrenal hemorrhage is typically self-limited with no sequelae.
- The appearance varies with the timing of imaging.
- Hemorrhage occurs more commonly on the right, but 10% of cases are bilateral.
- US: Appearance varies with age of the hemorrhage: acute—echogenic mass; subacute—mixed echotexture mass; chronic—may be calcified.
  - Serial US should demonstrate a retracting clot, with the adrenal gland eventually resuming its characteristic size and shape.

■ Other Imaging Findings

- Computed tomography: A nonenhancing suprarenal mass is dense if acute or hypodense if chronic.
- Magnetic resonance imaging: Appearance of aging blood products. Gradient echo will show blooming artifact.
- The hemorrhage may eventually calcify and can be seen as adrenal calcifications on subsequent studies (even years later).

✓ Pearls & ✗ Pitfalls

- ✓ Serial examinations demonstrate involution of the thrombus, differentiating it from an enlarging neuroblastoma.
- ✓ Ipsilateral renal vein thrombosis may coexist with the hemorrhage, particularly on the left.
- ✗ If serial US examinations do not demonstrate involution, magnetic resonance imaging should be performed to document blood products and rule out neuroblastoma.

Case 67

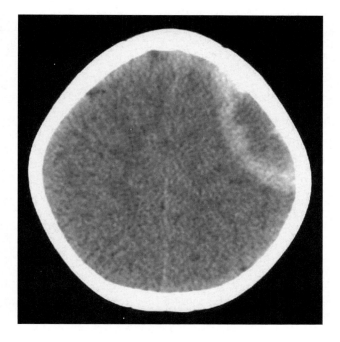

■ Clinical Presentation

A teenager who was involved in a high-speed motor vehicle collision.

■ Imaging Findings

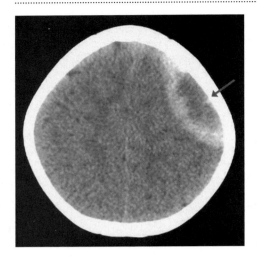

Axial noncontrast computed tomography (CT) image demonstrates a biconvex fluid collection along the left frontal lobe (*arrow*) exerting a considerable mass effect on the adjacent brain. The fact that the rim is bright but the central portion is isodense to brain suggests two distinct episodes of bleeding.

■ Differential Diagnosis

- *Epidural hematoma:* A lesion with a biconvex shape in the setting of recent head trauma is classic for epidural hematoma.
- *Subdural hematoma:* A subdural hematoma of this size would extend farther out along the lateral surface of the cerebral hemisphere because it is not bounded by sutures, and it therefore often exhibits a concave contour relative to the brain.
- *Cerebral contusion:* A cerebral contusion, centered in the brain parenchyma itself, could abut the inner table of the skull, but brain parenchyma should be seen interposed between the hematoma and the skull at both ends.

■ Essential Facts

- Epidural hematomas are seen most frequently in adolescents and young adults, who are most likely to be involved in high-impact trauma.
- Bleeding occurs in the potential space between the dura and the skull and is bounded by dural attachments to skull sutures.
- Approximately 90% result from damage to an artery, most commonly the middle meningeal artery.
- In 75 to 95% of cases, skull fractures are present.

✓ Pearls & ✗ Pitfalls

- ✓ Noncontrast CT is the imaging modality of choice for acute head trauma.
- ✓ Magnetic resonance imaging may be indicated if the CT findings are negative and epidural hematoma is strongly suspected clinically.
- ✓ Epidural hematoma may be associated with a "lucid interval," when the patient is conscious and alert, followed by deterioration with symptoms such as headache, vomiting, drowsiness, confusion, aphasia, seizures, and hemiparesis.

Case 68

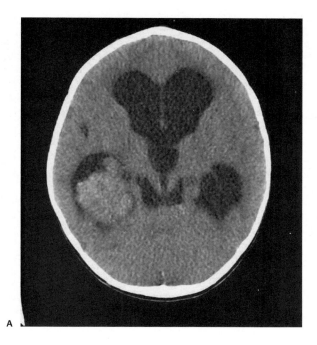

A

■ Clinical Presentation

An 8-month-old with an enlarging head circumference.

Further Work-up

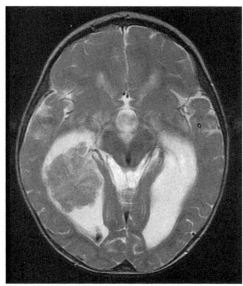

B

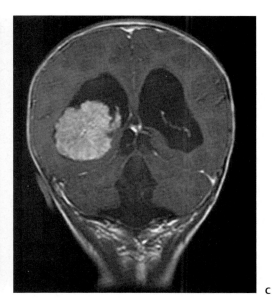

C

■ Imaging Findings

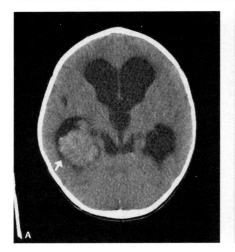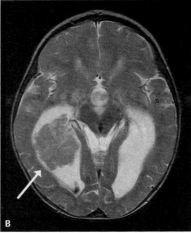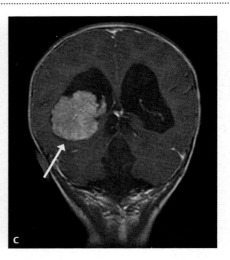

(A) Nonenhanced axial computed tomography image: there is a mildly hyperdense lobular mass in the right lateral ventricle (*arrow*), with enlargement of the lateral and third ventricles. **(B)** Axial T2 magnetic resonance image (MRI): there is a well-defined, lobular, isointense mass in the lateral ventricle (*arrow*), with enlargement of the ventricles. **(C)** Coronal T1 post-contrast MRI: there is marked enhancement of the mass (*arrow*).

■ Differential Diagnosis

- ***Choroid plexus papilloma (CPP)/carcinoma (CPCa):*** These findings are typical of CPP/CPCa.
- *Intraventricular hemorrhage:* Although an intraventricular hemorrhage can adhere to the choroid and appear mass-like, it would not enhance.
- *Sturge-Weber syndrome:* This causes enlargement of the choroid ipsilateral to a pial venous malformation. No other signs of Sturge-Weber syndrome are identified.

■ Essential Facts

- CPP/CPCa is a papillary neoplasm derived from choroid plexus epithelium.
- Most patients present before 5 years of age, with a marked male predominance.
- Patients present with signs and symptoms of elevated intracranial pressure.
- CPP/CPCa causes hydrocephalus secondary to the obstruction of ventricles, and rarely to the production of cerebrospinal fluid (CSF).
- The treatment is surgical excision.
- Five percent are cancerous.
- CPCa has a very poor prognosis.
- Perform contrast-enhanced MRI of the entire neuraxis before surgery to define the extent of disease.
- CPP and CPCa cannot be reliably distinguished by imaging. Both are lobulated, densely enhancing intraventricular masses that somewhat conform to the shape of the ventricle. One-fourth have calcification, and some have hemorrhage. CPCa may be necrotic.

- The most common location is the atria of the lateral ventricles (left > right); CPP and CPCa are less common in the 4th ventricle.
- Both may invade the brain and seed the CSF pathway.
- There may be flow voids within the mass.

✓ Pearls & ✗ Pitfalls

- ✓ Imaging cannot reliably distinguish between CPP and CPCa. Invasion into the brain parenchyma with heterogeneous enhancement and necrosis favors carcinoma.
- ✗ CPP and CPCa can occur in the 4th ventricle, but ependymoma and medulloblastoma are more common tumors of the 4th ventricle.

Case 69

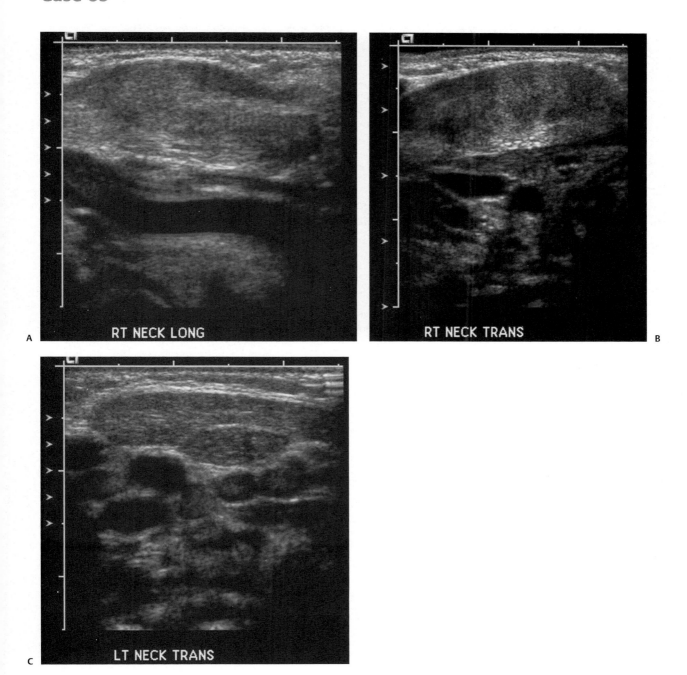

A — RT NECK LONG

B — RT NECK TRANS

C — LT NECK TRANS

■ Clinical Presentation

A 2-week-old boy with a firm mass in his neck and his head turned to the left.

■ Imaging Findings

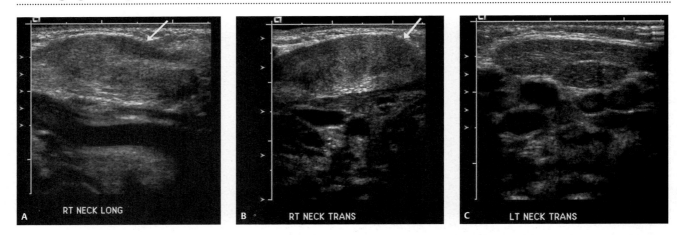

(A,B) Longitudinal and transverse ultrasound (US) images of the right side of the neck: The right sternocleidomastoid (SCM) muscle is enlarged (*arrows*). There is a subtle alteration of the echotexture in comparison with the normal left side. The fascial planes are intact. **(C)** Transverse US image of the left side of the neck: there is a normal-appearing left SCM muscle.

■ Differential Diagnosis

- **Fibromatosis colli:** These findings are typical of fibromatosis colli.
- *Cervical lymphadenopathy:* This usually has more of a lobulated contour with an echogenic/fatty hilum. A conglomeration of lymph nodes should have a more distorted architecture.
- *Branchial cleft anomalies:* These are usually cystic rather than solid and generally arise adjacent to the SCM muscle instead of within it.

■ Essential Facts

- Fibromatosis colli is likely due to perinatal injury, such as a partial muscle tear or intramuscular hematoma.
- Signs and symptoms include a painless, palpable mass and torticollis.
- Most often presents by 2 months of age and regresses spontaneously by 8 months; may increase in size after the initial presentation.
- If severe or persistent, fibromatosis colli can cause limited range of motion in the neck, as well as facial asymmetry.
- Treatment: In 90% of cases, patients have a full recovery with conservative treatment and/or physical therapy. Surgery is reserved for those with craniofacial asymmetry or refractory torticollis.
- The right side is affected more often than the left side.
- Focal thickening and fibrosis of the SCM muscle blends with the normal muscle. There should be intact fascial planes without inflammation or local invasion.
- US: Shows a well-marginated mass within the surrounding normal muscle, or diffuse enlargement of the muscle itself.

■ Other Imaging Findings

- Computed tomography/magnetic resonance imaging: The affected side should enhance symmetrically with the opposite side. These modalities are rarely needed.
- Plain films may be used to rule out other causes of torticollis, such as vertebral anomalies or omovertebral bones. On plain films, there may be nonspecific fullness, but fibromatosis colli almost never calcifies. Lytic lesions at the site of the muscular origins on the clavicle can occur.

✓ Pearls & ✗ Pitfalls

- ✓ When torticollis is involved, infants turn their head away from the affected side.
- ✗ Fibromatosis colli should be nontender. If the mass is tender, consider alternative diagnoses, such as infection or tumor.

Case 70

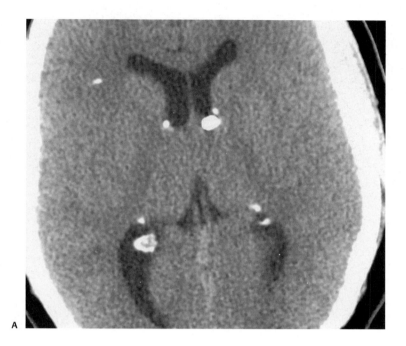

A

■ Clinical Presentation

A 10-year-old boy with seizures.

Further Work-up

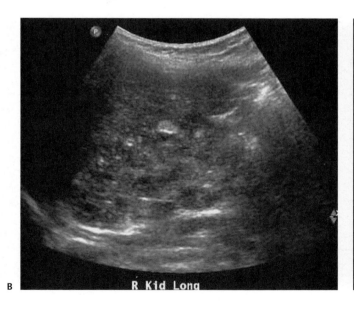

B   R Kid Long

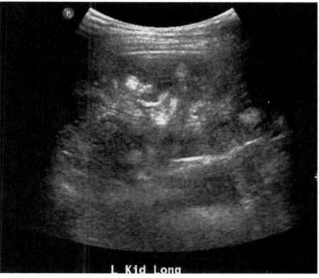

L Kid Long   C

■ Imaging Findings

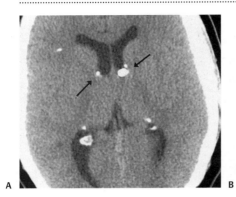 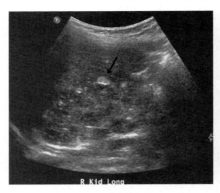 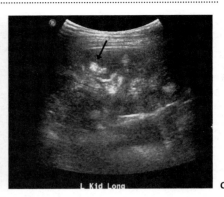

(A) Axial noncontrast computed tomography (CT) image: there are multiple calcified subependymal nodules (SENs, *arrows*). **(B,C)** Ultrasound images of the kidneys: there are multiple small hyperechoic nodules scattered throughout both kidneys (*arrows*).

■ Differential Diagnosis

- **Tuberous sclerosis:** Based on the calcified SENs and the echogenic lesions (angiomyolipomas) in the kidneys, this is the best diagnosis.
- *Sequela of a TORCH (toxoplasmosis, other infections, rubella, cytomegalovirus infection, herpes simplex) infection:* Cytomegalovirus (CMV) infection can have periventricular calcification; however, the calcifications on this study are subependymal. White matter lesions and polymicrogyria are also common in CMV infection and not seen here. Renal lesions are not consistent with CMV infection.
- *Gray matter heterotopia:* These lesions should have the same density as gray matter and do not calcify.

■ Essential Facts

- Multiorgan (central nervous system [CNS], skin, kidney, and bone) hamartomas are caused by a spontaneous or inherited tumor suppressor gene defect.
- If inherited, tuberous sclerosis is autosomal-dominant with high but variable penetrance.
- The classic clinical triad comprises facial angiofibromas, mental retardation, and seizures.
- Tuberous sclerosis can be diagnosed at any age because of the variable penetrance.
- CT
  - SENs: Calcification increases with time, so they may not be calcified in very young patients. Enlarging or enhancing SENs are a concern for subependymal giant cell astrocytoma (SGCA).
  - Tubers: These are hypo- or isodense subcortical masses that can be calcified.
- Typical findings include ventriculomegaly, calcified SENs, SGCA, cortical/subcortical tubers, and cystlike white matter lesions.

■ Other Imaging Findings

- Magnetic resonance imaging (MRI)
  - SEN enhancement is more prominent on MRI than on CT.
  - Tubers have increased T1 signal early, but this varies after myelin maturation.
  - Fluid attenuated inversion recovery images: Streaky or linear wedge-shaped hyperintensities are common as patients get older.

✓ Pearls & ✗ Pitfalls

- ✓ Associated non-CNS abnormalities include the following: renal angiomyolipomas and cysts, cardiac rhabdomyomas, retinal astrocytomas, giant ocular drusen, cystic lymphangiomyomatosis of the lungs, pigmentation defects in the skin, facial angiofibromas.
- ✗ An enlarging SEN at the foramen of Munro raises suspicion for SGCA.

Case 71

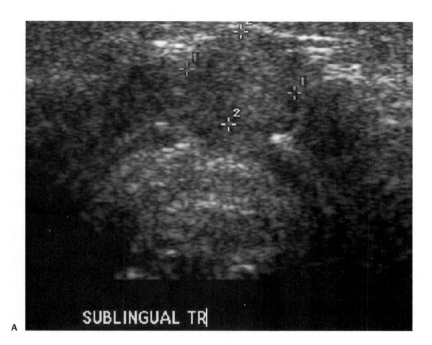

■ Clinical Presentation

An infant with a mass in the mouth.

Further Work-up

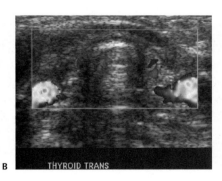

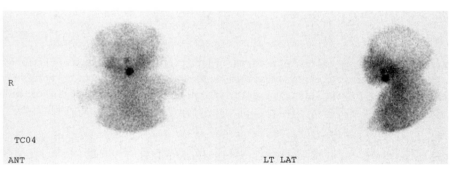

■ Imaging Findings

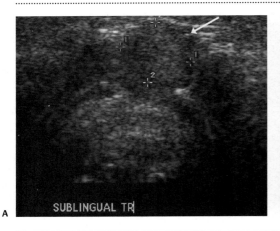
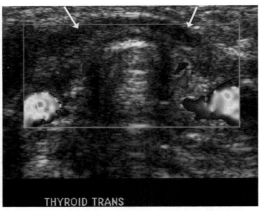
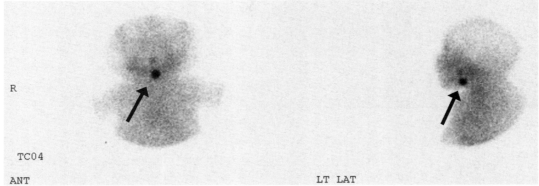

(A) Sublingual ultrasound (US) findings: there is a well-circumscribed, round, homogeneous mass (*arrow*). (B) Doppler US findings in the neck: there is no normal thyroid tissue in the thyroid bed (*arrows*). (C) Pertechnetate nuclear medicine study: there is uptake of pertechnetate at the base of the tongue (*arrows*).

■ Differential Diagnosis

- **Lingual thyroid:** An absence of normal thyroid tissue in the neck with a homogeneous mass at the base of the tongue that traps pertechnetate indicates lingual thyroid.
- *Thyroglossal duct cyst:* Would not trap pertechnetate. On US, it may be cystic but would have a solid component and possibly debris.
- *Enlarged lingual tonsil:* Would not trap pertechnetate.

■ Essential Facts

- Lingual thyroid is due to the arrested descent of normal thyroid from the base of the tongue between the 3rd and 7th week of gestation.
- When ectopic thyroid tissue is identified, thyroid function tests should be obtained to determine treatment.
- An ectopic thyroid may grow rapidly during puberty.
- Lingual thyroid appears as a well-circumscribed, round/ovoid mass at or near the midline at the base of the tongue.
- Ectopic thyroid can occur anywhere along the thyroglossal duct, from the base of the tongue to the thyroid bed.

■ Other Imaging Findings

- Computed tomography: On nonenhanced images, the ectopic thyroid gland has high density because of iodine. There is dense enhancement. If ectopic thyroid tissue is suspected, always comment on any thyroid tissue that may be present in the thyroid bed.
- Magnetic resonance imaging: T1 and T2 show increased signal compared with the tongue.

✓ Pearls & ✗ Pitfalls

- ✓ Lingual thyroid is the only functioning thyroid tissue in 75% of cases.
- ✗ In a nuclear imaging scan, pertechnetate is trapped by the thyroid but not organified. The uptake of pertechnetate demonstrates that the thyroid can trap iodine, but not necessarily incorporate it into functioning thyroid hormones.

Case 72

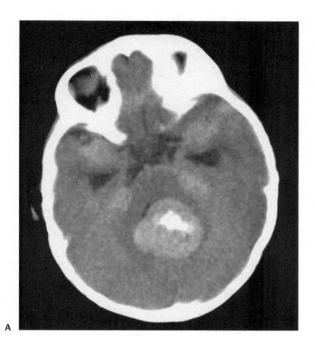

A

■ Clinical Presentation

A 3-year-old with ataxia.

Further Work-up

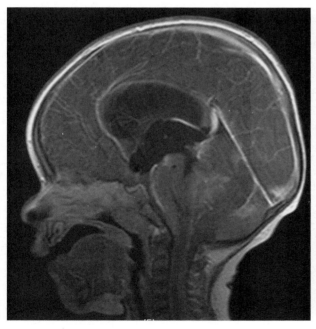

B

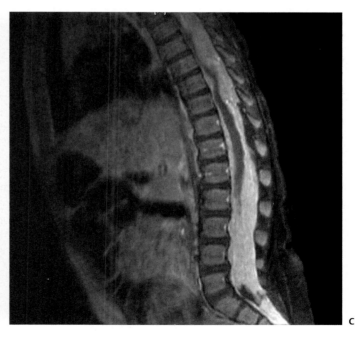

C

Imaging Findings

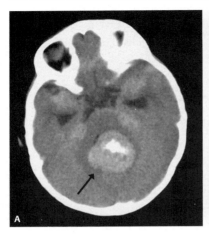 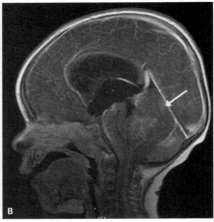 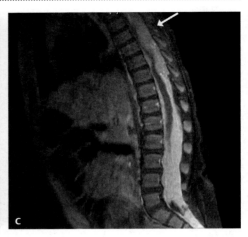

(A) Nonenhanced computed tomography (CT): there is a solid, hyperdense mass in the 4th ventricle with dense calcification (*arrow*). **(B)** Sagittal contrast-enhanced magnetic resonance image (MRI): there is an enhancing mass in the 4th ventricle (*arrow*) causing obstructive hydrocephalus. **(C)** Sagittal contrasted-enhanced MRI of the spine: there is extensive enhancing tumor within the spinal canal causing myelomalacia (*arrow*).

Differential Diagnosis

- **Medulloblastoma:** On CT, a hyperdense enhancing mass in the 4th ventricle with calcification and drop metastases to the spinal cord is likely a medulloblastoma.
- *Ependymoma:* Medulloblastoma and ependymoma can be difficult to differentiate. Ependymoma is usually a heterogeneous mass on CT that extends through the 4th ventricular foramina into the cisterns and arises from the floor of the 4th ventricle.
- *Pilocytic astrocytoma:* This is usually more cystlike with an enhancing mural nodule.

Essential Facts

- Medulloblastomas are primitive neuroectodermal tumors arising from the roof of the 4th ventricle.
- Most are diagnosed by 5 years of age, in boys more often than girls.
- There is a short duration of symptoms, which are caused by mass effect and increased intracranial pressure.
- The 5-year survival rate after complete resection, chemotherapy, and radiation is 40 to 80%. Recurrence is possible, usually within 3 to 5 years.
- A round, dense, intensely enhancing 4th ventricular mass tends to push away adjacent brain tissue rather than invade it.

Other Imaging Findings

- CT: 20% are calcified.
- MRI: On T1 they are hypointense to gray matter, and on T2 isointense to gray matter.
- Contrast-enhanced MRI of the entire neuraxis should be obtained to detect cerebrospinal fluid dissemination; may have linear enhancement over the brain surface.

✓ Pearls & ✗ Pitfalls

- ✓ Medulloblastomas can arise in a cerebellar hemisphere in older children.
- ✗ Medulloblastoma and ependymoma can be difficult to differentiate. Medulloblastomas arise from the roof of the 4th ventricle, whereas ependymomas arise from the floor of the 4th ventricle. Ependymomas are usually more heterogeneous and tend to calcify and hemorrhage more often.

Case 73

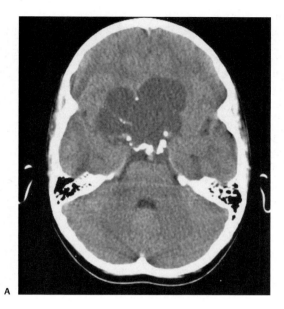

A

Clinical Presentation

A 10-year-old girl with headache and occasional vomiting.

Further Work-up

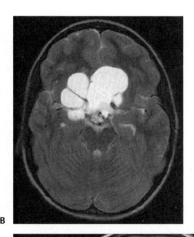

B

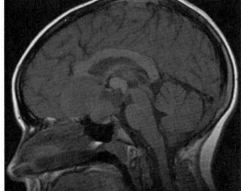

C

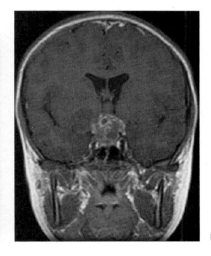

D

■ Imaging Findings

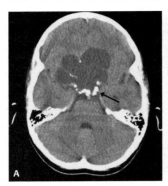 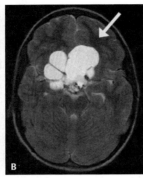 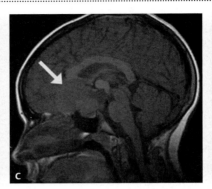 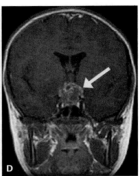

(A) Axial noncontrast computed tomography (CT) of the head: in the suprasellar region, there is a low-density, lobular mass with peripheral dense calcifications (*arrow*). **(B)** Axial T2-weighted magnetic resonance image (MRI): the lobular mass is fluid (*arrow*). **(C)** Sagittal T1-weighted MRI: the mass is intra- and suprasellar (*arrow*). **(D)** Coronal post-contrast MRI: there is peripheral enhancement (*arrow*).

■ Differential Diagnosis

- **Craniopharyngioma:** A cystic suprasellar mass with enhancing walls and calcifications is consistent with craniopharyngioma.
- *Rathke cleft cyst:* Usually does not enhance and has a solid component or calcifications.
- *Arachnoid cyst:* Has thin, nonenhancing walls, and the fluid portion follows cerebrospinal fluid on all sequences.

■ Essential Facts

- Craniopharyngioma is a slow-growing, benign tumor arising from squamous epithelial remnants along the Rathke duct (an embryonic tract between the pharynx and pituitary gland).
- The peak age is 5 to 12 years, but there is also an adult form that occurs in the 4th and 5th decades.
- Symptoms are due to mass effect on the optic chiasm and pituitary/hypothalamus, as well as elevated intracranial pressure.
- The treatment is surgical, but craniopharyngiomas tend to adhere to the adjacent brain structures, and surgery is often incomplete. Local recurrence is common, and radiotherapy is often necessary.
- A suprasellar mass has a large cystic component, a smaller solid component, and calcification, usually within the cyst wall. The solid component and cyst wall usually enhance.
- The tumor commonly extends outside the suprasellar region, causing obstructive hydrocephalus.
- CT 90% rule: 90% are cystic, 90% have calcifications, and 90% enhance.
- MRI: The cyst contents have variable signals due to protein, cholesterol, and blood components; often very bright on T1.

✓ Pearls & ✗ Pitfalls

- ✓ It is important to define the relationship of the tumor to the optic chiasm for planning surgery.
- ✓ This is the most common tumor of the suprasellar cistern.
- ✗ Rathke cleft cysts and small craniopharyngiomas can appear identical.

Case 74

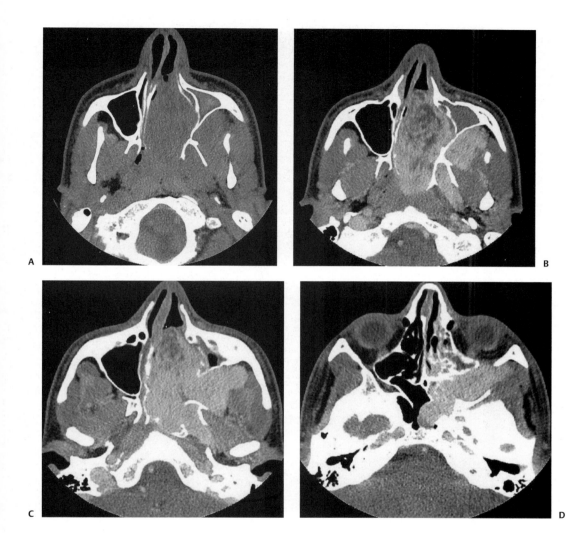

A

B

C

D

■ Clinical Presentation

A 15-year-old boy with nasal stuffiness.

Further Work-up

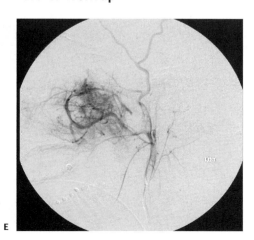

E

■ Imaging Findings

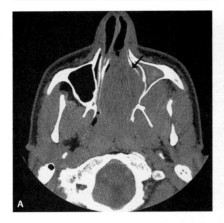 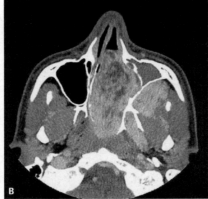 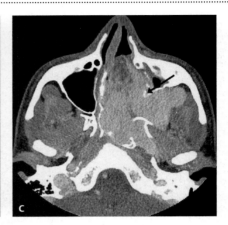

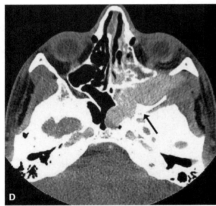 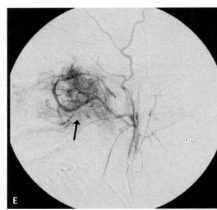

(A) Axial noncontrast computed tomography (CT): There is a soft-tissue mass filling the left nasal cavity and extending into the left nasopharynx (*arrow*). There is displacement of the posterior wall of the maxillary sinus and opacification of the maxillary sinus. **(B–D)** Axial contrast-enhanced CT images: there is dense contrast enhancement of the mass, which arises at the pterygopalatine fossa (PPF, *arrows*). **(E)** Anteroposterior digital subtraction external carotid arteriogram: there is a dense hypervascular tumor blush, with the major arterial supply from the distal left internal maxillary artery and its branches (*arrow*).

■ Differential Diagnosis

- *Juvenile nasopharyngeal angiofibroma (JNA):* These findings are typical of a JNA.
- *Rhabdomyosarcoma:* Would not have dense enhancement and does not generally involve the PPF or sphenopalatine foramen (SPF).
- *Polyp:* Would not involve the PPF or SPF and is not as densely enhancing.

■ Essential Facts

- JNA is a benign but aggressive nasopharyngeal tumor of mesenchymal origin.
- It is found nearly exclusively in 10- to 20-year-old males.
- Signs and symptoms include severe, often unilateral nosebleeds, airway obstruction, and recurrent middle ear disease.
- The treatment is complete surgical resection with preoperative embolization and/or steroids to minimize blood loss and reduce the size of the tumor. Radiation and hormonal therapy are controversial.
- There is a 25% rate of local recurrence after surgery.
- CT is excellent at defining bony detail; demonstrates mass at the SPF filling and enlarging the PPF; defines erosion of the pterygoid plate and displacement or erosion of the posterior wall of the maxillary sinus.

- A well-defined, densely enhancing mass involves the PPF and the SPF, with blood supply from the external carotid artery.

■ Other Imaging Findings

- Magnetic resonance imaging with fat saturation and contrast enhancement is best at detecting the intracranial extent of the tumor. On T1 and T2 images, multiple flow voids will be seen.
- Embolization can be performed during catheter angiography to minimize intraoperative blood loss.

✓ Pearls & ✗ Pitfalls

✓ JNA is a benign, aggressive, nonencapsulated hypervascular mass.

✓ It extends laterally into the PPF in 90% of cases.

✗ Biopsy in the outpatient setting should be avoided because of the risk for hemorrhage.

Case 75

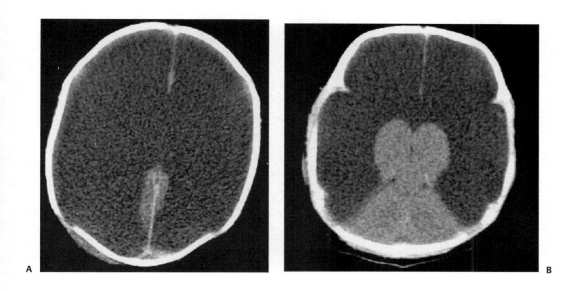

■ Clinical Presentation

A newborn with seizures.

■ Imaging Findings

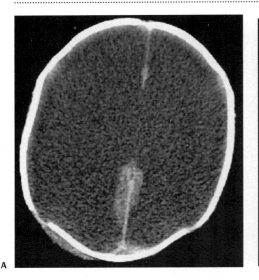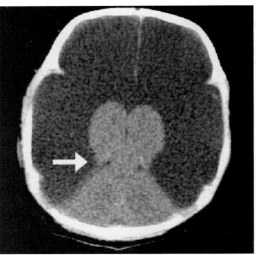

(A,B) Axial computed tomography images: There is absence of most of the cerebrum, with only a small amount of tissue along the falx. Cerebrospinal fluid (CSF) fills the cranial vault. The posterior fossa, thalami, and falx are intact (*arrow*).

■ Differential Diagnosis

- **Hydranencephaly:** An absent cerebrum with intact falx, thalami, and posterior fossa structures is consistent with hydranencephaly.
- *Alobar holoprosencephaly:* The falx would be absent and the midline structures would be fused.
- *Severe hydrocephalus:* A thin mantle of cortex would be seen surrounding the CSF.

■ Essential Facts

- Intrauterine compromise of the supraclinoid internal carotid arteries causes cerebral hemispheric destruction during gestation.
- Risk factors include thrombophilic states, intrauterine infection/anoxia, maternal irradiation/toxin exposure, and twin–twin transfusion.
- Hydranencephaly presents in the newborn with macrocrania, developmental failure, seizures, and hyperreflexia.
- Death occurs in infancy.
- Fluid fills most of the cranial vault. There is absence of the cerebrum; however, a small amount of tissue can remain along the inferior falx. The thalamus, brainstem, cerebellum, and choroid plexus are intact.

■ Other Imaging Findings

- Magnetic resonance imaging: the remaining brain has normal signal characteristics.

✓ Pearls & ✗ Pitfalls

- ✗ It can be very difficult to distinguish hydranencephaly from alobar holoprosencephaly, severe hydrocephalus, and severe bilateral schizencephaly.
  - Hydranencephaly has an intact falx, whereas alobar holoprosencephaly does not.
  - Hydrocephalus has a rim of tissue surrounding the enlarged ventricles, whereas hydranencephaly does not.
  - Schizencephaly has a gray matter–lined cleft, whereas hydranencephaly does not.

Case 76

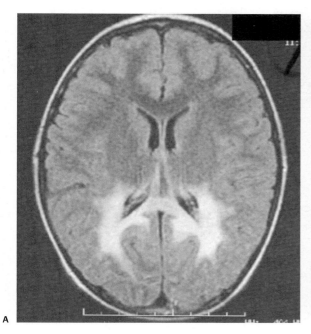
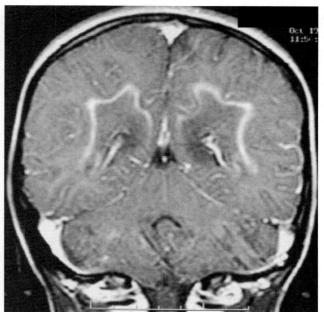

A B

■ Clinical Presentation

A 5-year-old boy with learning delays and gait abnormality.

■ Imaging Findings

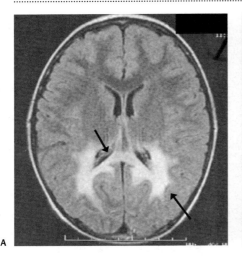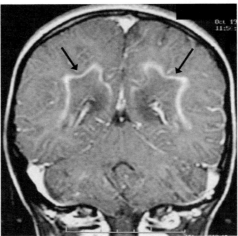

A   B

(A) Axial fluid-attenuated inversion recovery (FLAIR) image: there is abnormally high signal in the peritrigonal white matter and corpus callosum (*arrows*). **(B)** Coronal T1 post-contrast image: there is linear enhancement along the leading edge of the demyelination adjacent to the subcortical U-fibers (*arrows*).

■ Differential Diagnosis

- *X-linked adrenoleukodystrophy:* These findings are typical of adrenoleukodystrophy.
- *Posterior reversible encephalopathy syndrome:* This usually affects the cortical and subcortical regions in an asymmetric distribution and has variable patchy enhancement.
- *Periventricular leukomalacia:* Occurs after premature birth. Periventricular gliosis that does not enhance is associated with white matter volume loss and enlargement of the ventricles.

■ Essential Facts

- Adrenoleukodystrophy is an X-linked disorder of peroxisome metabolism affecting myelin formation and stabilization.
- It affects 5- to 10-year-old boys, but female carriers may show mild symptoms with a later onset.
- Classic signs and symptoms include behavioral/learning difficulties, hearing/vision problems, gait abnormalities, and signs of adrenal insufficiency (bronze skin, nausea, vomiting, fatigue).
- The condition progresses to spastic quadriparesis, blindness, deafness, and death in 2 to 5 years.
- Treatment: Bone marrow transplant may stop demyelination. Lorenzo's oil may prolong the time before symptoms develop. Other treatments have variable results.
- Usually, symmetric and confluent myelin degeneration begins in the occipital region, spreading anteriorly to involve the frontal lobes and corpus callosum and eventually the brainstem and cerebellum. Subcortical U-fibers are spared. Corticospinal tract involvement is fairly specific.

- The leading edge of myelin degeneration typically enhances (related to progression of disease).
- Magnetic resonance imaging: Involved white matter has a low signal on T1 and a high signal on T2 and FLAIR.

■ Other Imaging Findings

- Computed tomography: Decreased density is seen in the splenium of the corpus callosum and posterior white matter. Involved white matter can calcify.

✓ Pearls & ✗ Pitfalls

- ✓ Other leukodystrophies can have a similar appearance, with different distributions:
  - Metachromatic leukodystrophy: frontal and posterior with cerebellar involvement
  - Alexander disease: frontal predominance with subcortical white matter involvement
- ✗ There are at least six variants of adrenoleukodystrophy, some of which have different imaging characteristics. X-linked adrenoleukodystrophy is the most common.

Case 77

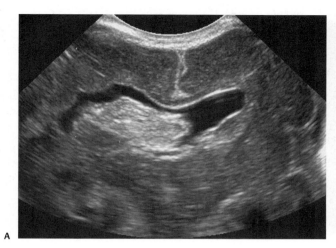
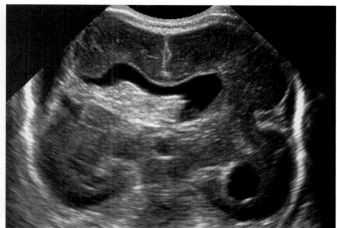

Clinical Presentation

A premature newborn with seizures.

Further Work-up

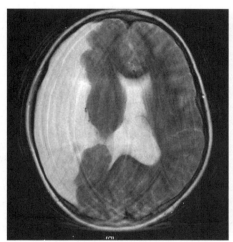
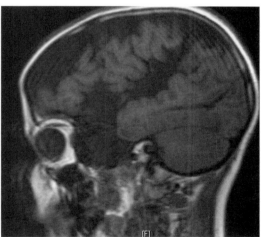

■ Imaging Findings

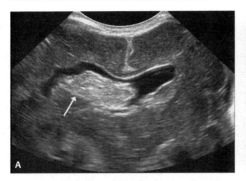 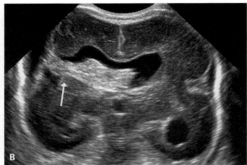 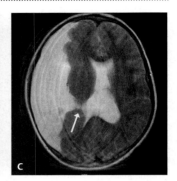

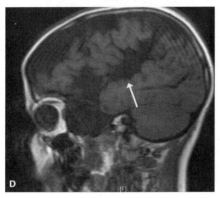

(A,B) Coronal ultrasound images: There is a cleft extending from the right lateral ventricle through the cortex to the extra-axial fluid. Choroid plexus extends through the cleft (*arrows*). Note the premature, smooth appearance of the brain and absence of the septum pellucidum. **(C)** Axial T2 MR image (several years later): again noted is a cleft extending from the lateral ventricle to the extra-axial fluid (*arrow*). **(D)** Sagittal T1 MR image (several years later): it is easier to tell on this image that the cleft is lined with gray matter (*arrow*).

■ Differential Diagnosis

- **Schizencephaly:** A cleft lined with gray matter extends from the ventricle through the cortex.
- *Porencephaly:* These defects are lined by gliotic white matter instead of gray matter.
- *Septo-optic dysplasia (SOD):* There is absence of the septum pellucidum; however, in SOD the clefts are usually bilateral. Furthermore, the optic nerves are not seen on these images.

■ Essential Facts

- A prenatal insult (maternal trauma, infection, or toxin exposure) or inherited mutation affects the germinal zone before neuronal migration.
- Patients with unilateral schizencephaly usually present with seizures and motor deficits, whereas those with bilateral schizencephaly usually have severe developmental delay, paresis, and spasticity.
- The severity of the defects determines the severity of impairment and treatment.
- A gray matter–lined cleft in the brain parenchyma extends from the ependyma to the pia.
- The most common location is in the frontal or parietal lobe near the central sulcus.
- There is a strong association with absence of the septum pellucidum and agenesis of the corpus callosum.

✓ Pearls & ✗ Pitfalls

- ✓ In closed-lip schizencephaly, the walls of the clefts touch. In open-lip schizencephaly, there is cerebrospinal fluid within the cleft.
- ✗ Visualization of the gray matter that lines the cleft can be difficult before myelination.
- ✗ The cleft can be easily overlooked if the plane of imaging is the same as the plane of the cleft. Multiplanar imaging helps avoid this problem.
- ✗ Closed-lip schizencephaly can be very subtle. Look for a dimple in the wall of the lateral ventricle.

Case 78

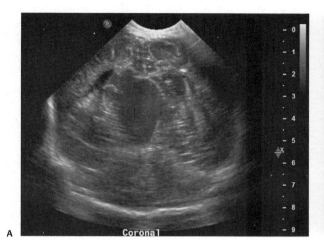

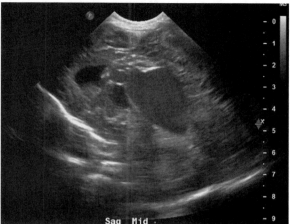

A Coronal   B Sag Mid

Clinical Presentation

Severe congestive heart failure in a full-term neonate. Ultrasound examination of the head was obtained to rule out intracranial hemorrhage before the patient was placed on extracorporeal membrane oxygenation.

Further Work-up

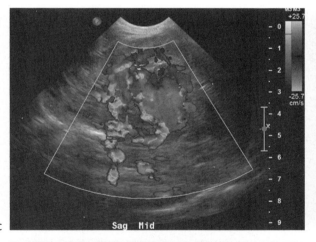

C Sag Mid

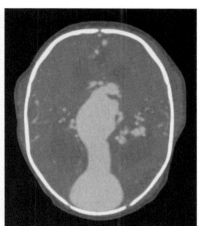

D

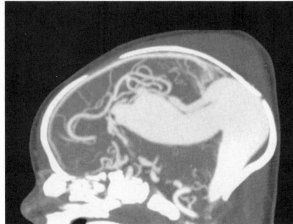

E

■ Imaging Findings

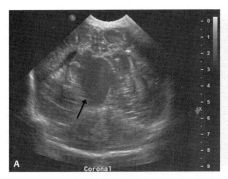 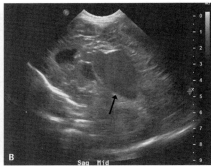 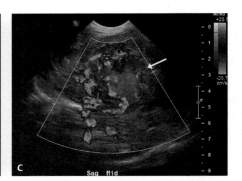

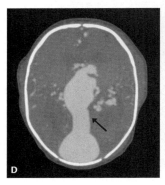 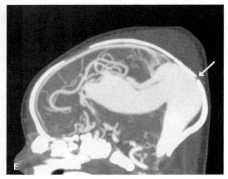

(A,B) Coronal and sagittal sonograms of the brain demonstrate a large, ovoid, cystic structure in the midline just posterior to the corpus callosum, in the expected location of the quadrigeminal plate cistern (*arrows*). **(C)** Sagittal Doppler ultrasound and **(D,E)** computed tomography angiography (CTA) images demonstrate that the structure contains flowing blood, consistent with an aneurysm (*arrows*).

■ Differential Diagnosis

- **Vein of Galen malformation:** In this clinical setting, the findings in a neonate of a large midline aneurysm in the region of the quadrigeminal plate cistern is virtually diagnostic.
- *True aneurysm:* A true aneurysm would not involve venous structures, whereas the vein of Galen malformation is associated with massive venous dilatation.
- *Choroid plexus cyst:* These lesions do not contain flowing blood and are not associated with heart failure.

■ Essential Facts

- Vein of Galen malformation is not really a venous malformation but an arteriovenous malformation (AVM), in which blood is carried straight from the deep choroidal arteries to a persistent vein of Markowski.
- The presence of the AVM prevents the formation of a normal vein of Galen.
- A high-volume left-to-right shunt means that much of the cardiac output simply returns to the heart without passing through a capillary bed or oxygenating tissues, forcing the heart to work much harder to maintain adequate tissue oxygenation.

- In patients who present with heart failure, the mortality rate is very high.
- Vein of Galen malformation is often associated with a cranial bruit.

✓ Pearls & ✗ Pitfalls

- ✓ Magnetic resonance angiography and CTA can provide accurate vessel mapping, with conventional angiography reserved for intervention.
- ✓ Although success rates are mixed, embolization is becoming the treatment of choice.

Case 79

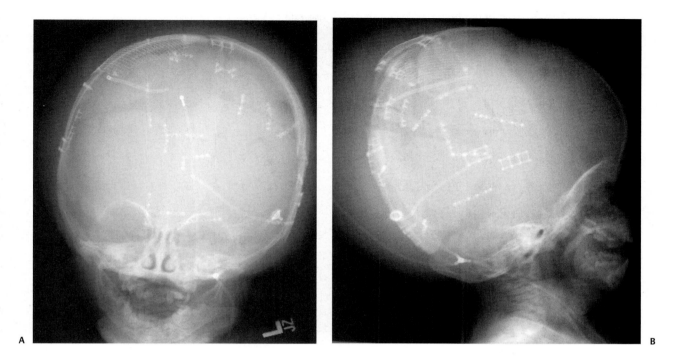

A   B

■ Clinical Presentation

A toddler who previously underwent craniotomy and ventriculoperitoneal shunting during resection of a brain tumor presents with headache and a posterior head mass.

■ Imaging Findings

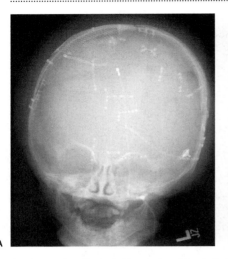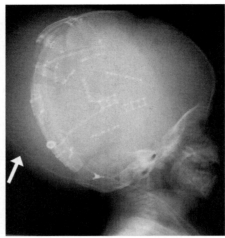

(A,B) Frontal and lateral radiographs of the skull obtained as part of a ventriculoperitoneal shunt series demonstrate a large, crescentic soft-tissue mass along the back of the skull, as well as disruption of the shunt catheter, a portion of which extends posterior to the mass (*arrow*).

■ Differential Diagnosis

- ***Disrupted shunt catheter:*** The finding of a soft-tissue mass adjacent to a disconnected segment of shunt catheter is strongly suggestive of a collection of cerebrospinal fluid ("CSFoma"), which results from leakage of CSF that should be traveling down the catheter into the peritoneal cavity.
- *Abandoned shunt catheter:* In this situation, an unattached segment of catheter does not indicate disruption because a second shunt catheter is now functioning to drain CSF, or the patient no longer requires shunting. Moreover, abandoned shunt catheters should not be associated with CSF collections presenting as soft-tissue masses.
- *Pseudo-disruption:* Some swelling is normal in the periop-erative period after catheter placement, and many cath-eters exhibit radiolucent segments that can be mistaken for disruptions.

■ Essential Facts

- Approximately 125,000 patients in the United States have a ventriculoperitoneal shunt, placed to relieve hydrocepha-lus.
- Causes of hydrocephalus include increased CSF production (choroid plexus papilloma), obstruction to CSF flow (tumor or congenital stenosis), and impaired venous resorption (meningitis or subarachnoid hemorrhage).
- Common symptoms and signs of increased intracranial pressure are headache (especially in the morning, with nausea and vomiting), mood changes, bulging of the fonta-nelles, increased head circumference, and papilledema.

■ Other Imaging Findings

- Ultrasound (US) is the initial imaging modality to assess for hydrocephalus in infants.
- US can also be used to follow the size of CSF spaces over time, before and after shunting.
- Computed tomography and magnetic resonance imaging provide greater anatomic detail.

✓ Pearls & ✗ Pitfalls

- ✓ Causes of ventriculoperitoneal shunt malfunction include infection, valve failure, disruption of the catheter, and clogging, among other possibilities.
- ✓ If the shunt is intact, contrast injection may be warranted to confirm catheter patency.

Case 80

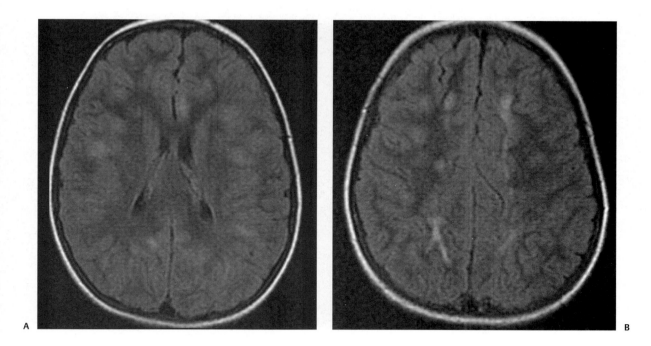

A

B

■ Clinical Presentation

A 7-year-old with inability to walk after a recent viral illness.

Further Work-up

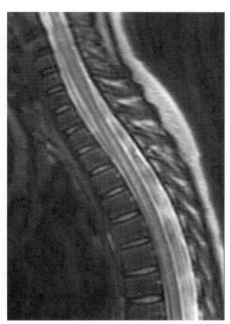

C

■ **Imaging Findings**

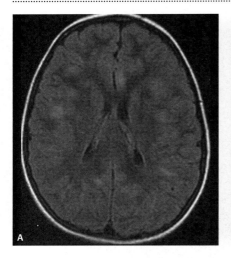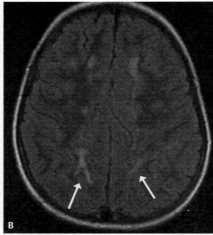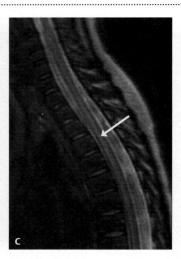

(A,B) Axial fluid-attenuated inversion recovery (FLAIR) magnetic resonance images (MRIs): there are bilaterally asymmetric, patchy, high-signal areas in the gray matter and subcortical white matter (*arrows*). **(C)** Sagittal T2 image of the thoracic spine: there are abnormal areas of increased signal in the central portion of the cord (*arrow*).

■ **Differential Diagnosis**

- *Acute disseminated encephalomyelitis (ADEM):* These lesions are characteristic of ADEM.
- *Multiple sclerosis (MS):* ADEM and MS lesions can appear identical, but MS lesions are usually more regular in shape and more symmetric.
- *Posterior reversible encephalopathy syndrome:* Usually, only the posterior cerebral artery territory and watershed areas are affected. The spinal cord is not involved.

■ **Essential Facts**

- The peak age is 3 to 5 years.
- ADEM usually occurs 1 to 2 weeks after a viral infection or vaccination.
- Signs and symptoms include headache, cranial nerve palsies, seizures, hemiparesis, and decreased consciousness.
- The condition is most commonly monophasic, with complete recovery within 1 month in half of cases. Neurologic sequelae (usually seizures) develop in 20 to 30% of patients.
- The treatment includes steroids, immunoglobulin, and plasmapheresis.
- Amorphous, sometimes spherical/ovoid lesions are typically small and multifocal, without mass effect.
- Lesions have a predilection for the subcortical white matter but are also found in the basal ganglia and some gray matter. The cerebrum is affected more often than the cerebellum.
- MRI: Lesions appear bright on T2 and FLAIR images. Post-contrast images may show punctate or ring enhancement. Cranial nerves may enhance.

■ **Other Imaging Findings**

- Computed tomography: Noncontrast—lesions have low density. Post-contrast—more lesions are usually identified.

✓ **Pearls & ✗ Pitfalls**

✓ Imaging findings may lag behind the symptoms. Initial studies may be negative.

✗ It is difficult to distinguish between MS and ADEM, but MS has a relapsing-remitting course.

Case 81

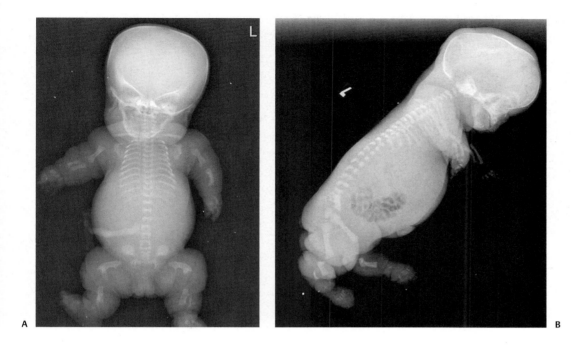

Clinical Presentation

A stillborn dysmorphic infant.

■ Imaging Findings

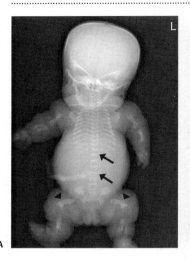
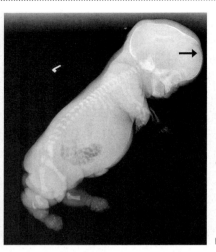

(A) Frontal "babygram" demonstrates extremely short ribs with associated pulmonary hypoplasia, platyspondyly (flat vertebral bodies, *arrows*), and micromelic shortening of all the long bones, with "telephone receiver" femora (*arrowheads*). **(B)** Lateral view demonstrates frontal bossing (*arrow*) and better shows the extreme flattening of the vertebral bodies and limb shortening.

■ Differential Diagnosis

- **Thanatophoric dysplasia:** The extreme shortening of the ribs and long bones, flattening of the vertebral bodies, and telephone receiver shape of the femora are characteristic of this disorder.
- *Achondroplasia:* This is associated with less severe shortening of the ribs and long bones, is not associated with platyspondyly or telephone receiver femora, and is generally not lethal at birth.
- *Mucopolysaccharidoses:* These cause less severe dwarfism, are generally not lethal at birth, and are associated with lumbar gibbous deformity and vertebral beaking.

■ Essential Facts

- The name is derived from the Greek words *thanatos* ("death") and *pherein* ("to carry, bear")—thus "bringing death."
- This is the most common form of lethal skeletal dysplasia.
- It is associated with an autosomal-dominant sporadic mutation in *FGFR3*, the same gene that causes achondroplasia.
- Type 1 characteristics include the following:
  - Macrocephaly
  - Micromelic shortening of limbs
  - Frontal bossing
  - Bell-shaped abdomen
- Type 2 characteristics include the following:
  - Clover-leaf skull and premature closure of sutures
  - Straight femora

✓ Pearls & ✗ Pitfalls

- ✓ In infants who survive, neuroimaging is recommended to assess for ventriculomegaly, craniosynostosis, and stenosis of the foramen magnum.

Case 82

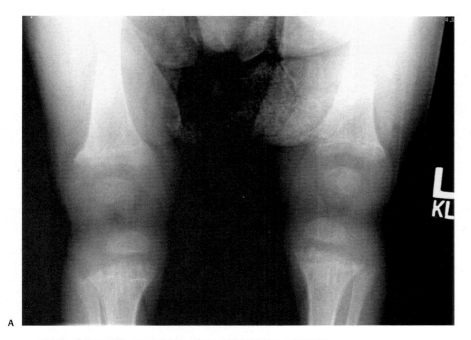

A

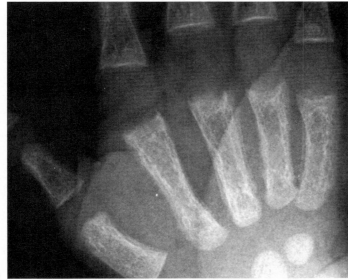

B

■ Clinical Presentation
....

A toddler with bowed legs.

◼ Imaging Findings

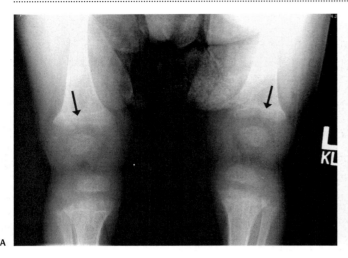
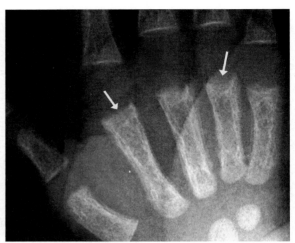

(A) Frontal radiographs of both knees demonstrate cupping and fraying of the metaphyses of the long bones (*arrows*), widening of the physes, and diffuse osteopenia. **(B)** A radiograph of the patient's hand, which is not necessary for diagnosis, demonstrates cupping and fraying of the metaphyses of the metacarpals (*arrows*) with subperiosteal linear lucencies.

◼ Differential Diagnosis

- *Rickets:* The cupping and fraying of the metaphyses, widening of the growth plates, osteopenia, and clinical history of bowed legs are typical of rickets.
- *Leukemia:* Lucent metaphyseal bands can mimic widening of the growth plates, and some patients may be osteopenic, but the cupping and fraying of the metaphyses and the history of bowing do not fit.
- *Syphilis:* Patients with congenital syphilis may have lucent metaphyseal bands, but the cupping and fraying are not features of syphilis, which often demonstrates resorption of the medial aspects of the proximal tibial metaphyses, not seen in this case.

◼ Essential Facts

- The incidence of rickets is low in the United States, but the disease occurs in darker-skinned children, lactovegans, and persons with malabsorptive syndromes, chronic renal failure, or metabolic disorders.
- Rickets is associated with a deficiency of vitamin D, calcium, or phosphorus, all of which are necessary for normal bone development.
- Softening of the skull (craniotabes) can result in postural molding.
- Cupping of the anterior rib ends can produce the "rachitic rosary."

✓ Pearls & ✗ Pitfalls

- ✓ In young children, the distal ulna is the most sensitive bone, whereas in older children, the knee is the most sensitive.
- ✓ Bowing is most severe in the hypophosphatemic form.
- ✓ Rickets became fairly common during the industrial revolution, likely representing the first childhood disease associated with environmental pollution.

Case 83

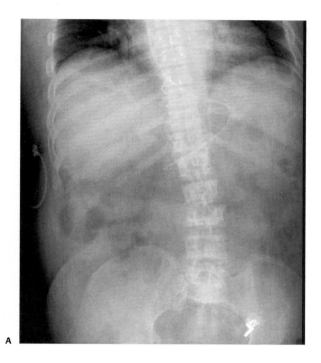

A

■ Clinical Presentation

A child with painful scoliosis.

Further Work-up

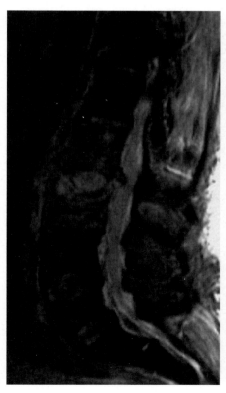

B

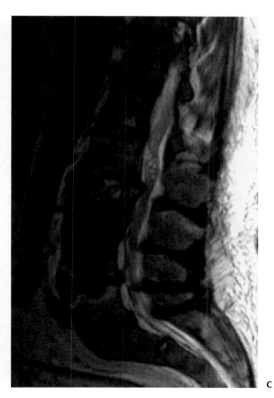

C

■ Imaging Findings

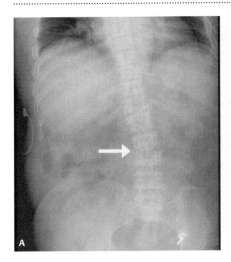 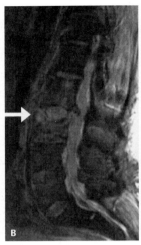 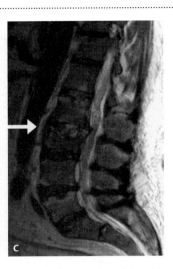

(A) Frontal abdominal radiograph demonstrates levoscoliosis of the lumbar spine associated with narrowing of the L2-3 intervertebral disk space and possible destruction of the end plates of the adjacent vertebrae (*arrow*). **(B,C)** Sagittal T2 and T1 post-contrast magnetic resonance images (MRIs) of the lumbar spine demonstrate destruction of the intervertebral disk and adjacent vertebral end plates with abnormally increased signal and enhancement (*arrows*), as well as herniation of the disk contents into the vertebral canal.

■ Differential Diagnosis

- **Diskitis:** The plain radiographic findings of intervertebral disk space narrowing and end plate irregularity, as well as MRI findings of disk and end plate inflammation and destruction, are diagnostic.
- *Neoplasm:* Involvement of the spine by Langerhans cell histiocytosis or leukemia, as well as metastatic processes such as neuroblastoma, can cause vertebral body destruction, but the process should not be centered at the intervertebral disk.
- *Scheuermann disease:* Disk space narrowing and end plate irregularity are features of this disorder, but it involves at least three vertebral body levels, is associated with kyphosis, and usually occurs in the thoracic spine. Inflammation is not a feature on MRI.

■ Essential Facts

- Diskitis is most common between infancy and the age of 3 years, although it is possible in adolescence.
- The typical presentation includes irritability, back pain, refusal to walk, and fever in 25%.
- Many cases are thought to be aseptic and resolve without antibiotics.
- Diskitis occurs most commonly in the lumbar spine.
- Plain radiographic findings may be normal for 2 weeks, showing only narrowing of the intervertebral spaces. Later, the radiograph shows the following:
  - Irregularities and erosion of the adjacent end plates
  - Calcification of the annulus around the affected disk
  - Decreased bone density, with loss of the normal trabeculation of the vertebra
  - Subluxation, which becomes evident with further osteolysis

- MRI is the test of choice for the diagnosis because it is the most sensitive and specific:
  - T1-weighted images show narrowing of the disk space and low signal, consistent with edema in the marrow of adjacent vertebral bodies.
  - T2-weighted images show increased signal in both the disk space and the surrounding vertebral bodies.
  - The disk space pattern helps rule in diskitis and rule out tuberculosis and neoplasm.
  - MRI is excellent for visualizing pathology in the paraspinal tissues.

■ Other Imaging Findings

- Computed tomography is more sensitive than plain radiograph and may show the following:
  - Hypodensity of the intervertebral disk
  - Destruction of the adjacent end plate and bone with edematous surrounding tissues
  - Gas from bacteria and other soft-tissue changes
  - Sclerosis and increased bone density on follow-up, indicating improvement
- Bone scan is very sensitive early, but MRI provides more anatomic detail.

✓ Pearls & ✗ Pitfalls

- ✓ Plain radiographs are often negative until symptoms have been present for 2 weeks.
- ✓ MRI is most sensitive and specific, particularly early in the course of disease.

Case 84

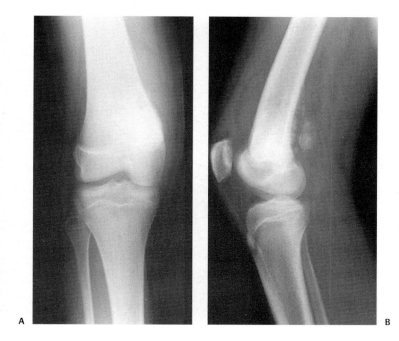

A

B

■ Clinical Presentation

A teenager with knee pain.

■ Imaging Findings

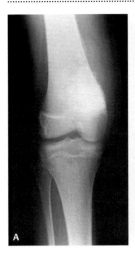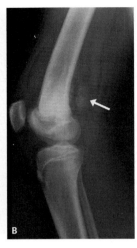

(A,B) Lateral and frontal radiographs of the knee demonstrate an aggressive periosteal reaction along the distal femoral metaphysis, associated with a Codman triangle, soft-tissue mass, and cloudlike osteoid matrix, best seen posterior to the femoral metaphysis on the lateral view (*arrow*).

■ Differential Diagnosis

- ***Osteosarcoma:*** The distal femoral location, aggressive periosteal reaction, soft-tissue mass, and osteoid matrix are all typical of osteosarcoma.
- *Ewing sarcoma:* The other common primary bone malignancy in children and teenagers, Ewing sarcoma is relatively more common in the diaphyses and not associated with an osteoid matrix.
- *Osteomyelitis:* This can be associated with both bone lysis and sclerosis, but the cellular process is incapable of producing new bone matrix.

■ Essential Facts

- Osteosarcoma is the most common primary bone malignancy of childhood and young adulthood.
- Nearly half of cases involve the femur, with the tibia, humerus, pelvis, skull, and jaw less commonly affected.
- The typical presentation is a painful mass.

■ Other Imaging Findings

- Magnetic resonance imaging is indicated to assess the extent of the lesion and detect "skip" lesions.
- Bone scan is indicated to assess for involvement of other bones.
- Chest computed tomography is indicated to evaluate for pulmonary metastasis.

✓ Pearls & ✗ Pitfalls

- ✓ Nearly half of lesions are osteoblastic, a third are osteolytic, and the remainder are mixed.
- ✓ A "sunburst" pattern indicates tumor "exploding" outward through the periosteum.

Case 85

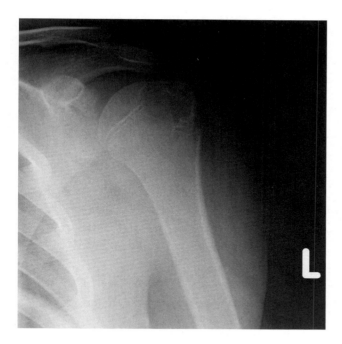

▦ Clinical Presentation

A preteen with shoulder pain.

■ Imaging Findings

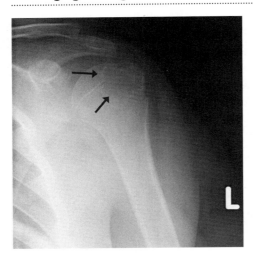

Frontal radiograph of the shoulder demonstrates a lytic lesion in the proximal humeral epiphysis, with no evidence of fracture or periosteal reaction (*arrows*). The lesion does not cross the growth plate.

■ Differential Diagnosis

- **Chondroblastoma:** The epiphyseal origin, eccentric location, lytic appearance, and sharp borders are all typical.
- *Giant cell tumor:* The location and lytic appearance are not atypical, but giant cell tumors are almost never seen in skeletally immature patients.
- *Osteomyelitis:* Can have an identical appearance, although often accompanied by other symptoms and signs of infection. Biopsy is often necessary to distinguish osteomyelitis from chondroblastoma.

■ Essential Facts

- Ninety percent occur in persons between 5 and 25 years of age, with a 3:1 male predominance.
- Chondroblastoma typically presents with pain, tenderness, and swelling.
- One-third of patients have a joint effusion.
- Three-fourths involve the lower extremity, and half are at the knee.
- Nearly half are uniformly lucent, but others have a mottled appearance.

■ Other Imaging Findings

- Computed tomography may show a chondroid matrix, fluid-fluid levels, and septation.
- Magnetic resonance imaging typically shows a low T1 signal, a high/mixed T2 signal, and fluid-fluid levels.

✓ Pearls & ✗ Pitfalls

- ✓ Consider this diagnosis for a lucent lesion in an apophysis.
- ✓ When present at the hip, chondroblastoma tends to involve the greater trochanter more commonly than the capital femoral epiphysis.
- ✓ Recurrence after surgical resection is seen in up to one-third of cases.

Case 86

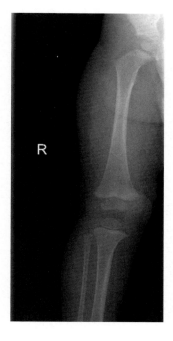

■ Clinical Presentation

A toddler who refuses to bear weight on the right leg.

■ Imaging Findings

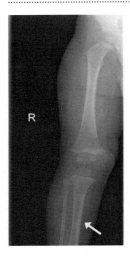

Frontal radiograph of the femur demonstrates an oblique lucency extending through the diaphysis of the tibia, consistent with spiral fracture (*arrow*).

■ Differential Diagnosis

- **Toddler fracture:** The clinical presentation and oblique lucency are classic for toddler fracture.
- *Osteomyelitis/septic arthritis:* This also presents with refusal to bear weight, but local and systemic signs of infection should be present, and no fracture will be apparent.
- *Toxic synovitis:* Plain radiographic findings are normal, with the possible exception of a hip joint effusion, which is better visualized on ultrasound.

■ Essential Facts

- This is also called the toddler's fracture, or childhood accidental spiral tibia fracture.
- The mean age is higher than originally thought: approximately 50 months.
- Toddler fracture results from a jerking, twisting motion of the limb, as in turning quickly to look at something.
- It is not associated with bruising or deformity.
- Pain occurs on gentle twisting of the tibia.

■ Other Imaging Findings

- Fracture is apparent on bone scan as increased uptake after 2 days.
- Computed tomography can demonstrate fracture immediately.
- Magnetic resonance imaging shows fracture as a hypointense linear lucency with surrounding marrow hemorrhage and edema.

✓ Pearls & ✗ Pitfalls

✓ When frontal and lateral views do not demonstrate fracture, an oblique plain radiograph is often diagnostic.

Case 87

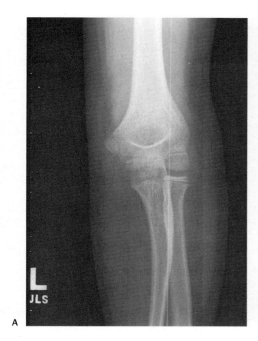
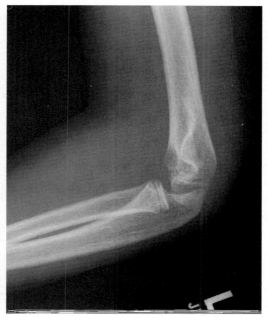

A   B

■ Clinical Presentation

Elbow pain after trauma.

■ Imaging Findings

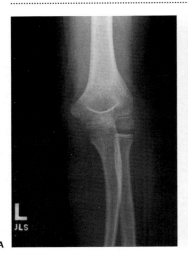 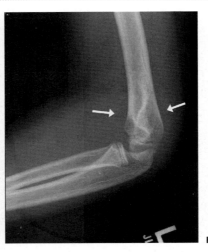

(A) Frontal radiograph of the elbow demonstrates mild soft-tissue swelling but no fracture. **(B)** Lateral radiograph of the elbow demonstrates prominent anterior and posterior fat pads (*arrows*), which in this setting are highly suggestive of a supracondylar fracture.

■ Differential Diagnosis

- ***Supracondylar fracture:*** Prominent fat pad signs in the setting of acute elbow trauma without radiographically apparent fracture are typical of occult supracondylar fracture.
- *Avascular necrosis of the capitellum:* This is most common in teenagers involved in gymnastics and throwing.
- *Arthritis:* Juvenile arthritis can present with elbow pain and effusion, although the symptoms are not traceable to a single episode of trauma.

■ Essential Facts

- Supracondylar fracture is the most common pediatric elbow fracture.
- The peak incidence is between 5 and 10 years.
- Ninety-five percent involve a disruption of the anterior cortex, often not apparent radiographically in the acute setting.
- The distal humerus is most fragile in its midportion, between the medial and lateral columns, which flare out to form the condyles.

✓ Pearls & ✗ Pitfalls

- ✓ A positive fat pad sign warrants presumptive treatment for a fracture, and the fracture line itself often becomes visible on subsequent imaging.

Case 88

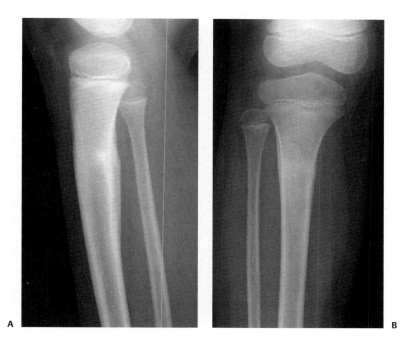

A

B

■ Clinical Presentation

Persistent calf pain in an athlete.

Further Work-up

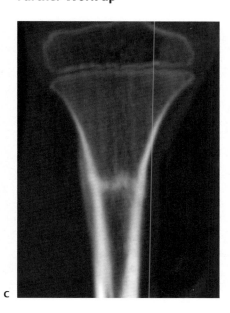

C

◼ Imaging Findings

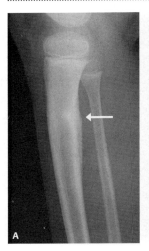
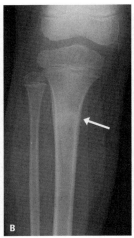
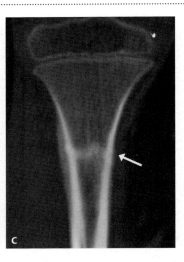

(A,B) Frontal and lateral plain radiographs of the proximal tibia and fibula demonstrate a transverse band of sclerosis extending across the proximal tibia, with an associated periosteal reaction (*arrows*). **(C)** Coronal reformat computed tomography image of the proximal tibia again demonstrates the transverse sclerosis and periosteal reaction of the proximal tibia (*arrow*).

◼ Differential Diagnosis

- **Tibial stress fracture:** The transverse sclerosis and posterior location are typical.
- *Osteoid osteoma:* Often associated with pain that is worse at night and relieved by nonsteroidal anti-inflammatory medications. The classic imaging appearance is that of a sclerotic lesion with a lucent nidus that should not be so transversely oriented.
- *Brodie abscess:* This may also appear as a sclerotic lesion with a lucent nidus, although again not typically transversely oriented.

◼ Essential Facts

- Tibial stress fracture is most common in children who have recently increased their physical activity/sports training.
- The mechanism is repetitive loading while the bone is temporarily weakened by resorption in preparation for remodeling.
- Stress fracture most commonly affects the proximal tibia, fibula, vertebral pars interarticularis, and femur.
- The typical presentation involves initial pain with exercise, then improvement with rest, but the pain will become more constant if the patient persists in activity.

◼ Other Imaging Findings

- In the acute setting, magnetic resonance imaging (MRI) is the test of choice, demonstrating linear hypointensity extending transversely across the bone, with surrounding edema.
- Scintigraphy may be helpful if MRI is contraindicated or unavailable.

✓ Pearls & ✗ Pitfalls

✓ Plain radiographic findings may not be positive for 1 to 2 weeks.

Case 89

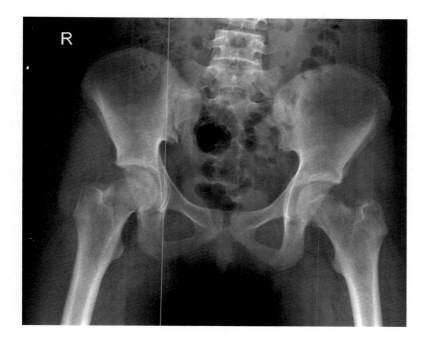

■ Clinical Presentation

A teenage athlete with acute hip pain following exertion.

■ Imaging Findings

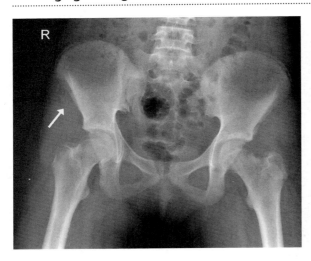

Frontal radiograph of the pelvis demonstrates a sliver of bone (*arrow*) lateral to the right anterior superior iliac spine.

■ Differential Diagnosis

- ***Avulsion fracture of the anterior superior iliac spine:*** The finding of a fragment of bone adjacent to a muscular attachment in this clinical setting is essentially pathognomonic.
- *Acute fracture:* Acute fractures about the hip are generally associated with collisions, not mere exertion.
- *Slipped capital femoral epiphysis:* This is more common in obese patients and associated with widening of the proximal femoral physis.

■ Essential Facts

- Avulsion fracture of the anterior superior iliac spine is most common in young athletes, often runners who exert great force in extending a leg.
- The fractures generally heal completely with rest.
- Surgery may be required to restore anatomic fixation or remove painful fragments.

✓ Pearls & ✗ Pitfalls

- ✓ The anterior superior iliac spine is the attachment point of the sartorius and tensor fasciae latae muscles.
- ✓ The anterior inferior iliac spine is the attachment point of the rectus femoris, and the ischial tuberosity attaches the hamstrings.

Case 90

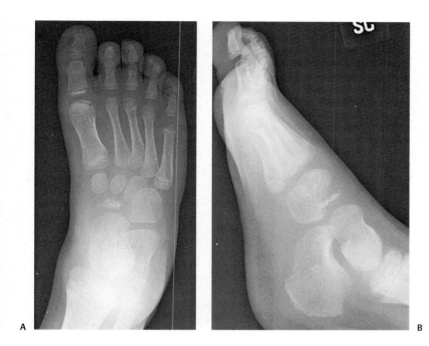

A

B

Clinical Presentation

A 3-year-old boy with a limp and pain and tenderness over the medial aspect of his right foot.

■ Imaging Findings

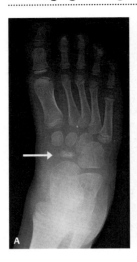 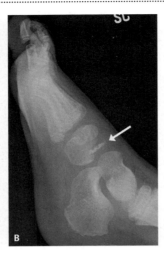

(A,B) Lateral and frontal radiographs of the right foot demonstrate flattening and sclerosis of the tarsal navicular bone (*arrows*).

■ Differential Diagnosis

- **Kohler disease:** Flattening and sclerosis of the navicular are typical findings.
- *Normal:* Irregular ossification of the navicular can be normal, and the diagnosis of this relatively uncommon condition should be considered only in symptomatic patients.
- *Osteomyelitis:* A rare condition in this location that should be accompanied by local and systemic signs of infection.

■ Essential Facts

- This disease was first described by Alban Kohler, a German radiologist, in 1908.
- It is more common in boys than girls, with a peak age of 5 years.
- Kohler disease is one of the osteochondroses, likely due to repetitive microtrauma with avascular necrosis.
- The treatment is nonsurgical, with resolution of the symptoms in weeks and a normal appearance of the navicular in months.

✓ Pearls & ✗ Pitfalls

- ✓ The tarsal navicular is the last bone in the foot to ossify.
- ✓ The treatment is nonsurgical.

Case 91

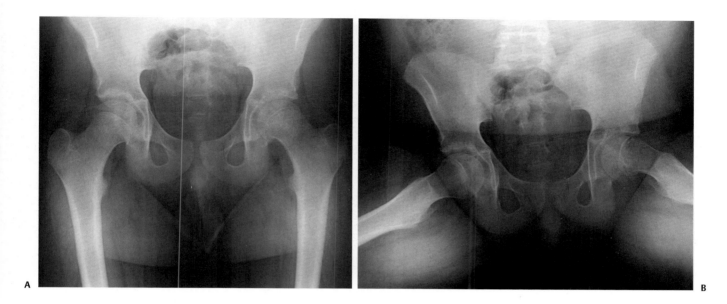

■ Clinical Presentation

A preadolescent boy with left hip pain.

■ Imaging Findings

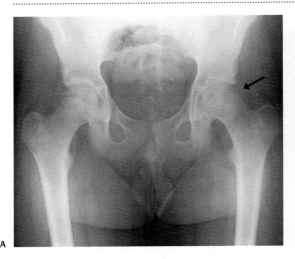
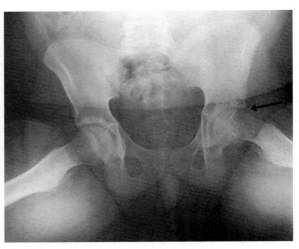

A   B

(A,B) Frontal and frog-leg radiographs of the pelvis demonstrate a widened proximal femoral growth plate on the left, with lateral displacement of the left femoral metaphysis relative to the epiphysis (*arrows*).

■ Differential Diagnosis

- **Slipped capital femoral epiphysis:** The widening of the physis and lateral displacement of the metaphysis relative to the epiphysis are typical.
- *Perthes disease:* This generally occurs between 5 and 10 years of age and should demonstrate a normal relationship between the femoral metaphysis and epiphysis, with signs of avascular necrosis in the femoral epiphysis.
- *Arthritis:* This is associated with hip joint effusion and accompanied by systemic symptoms of infection or a rheumatologic condition.

■ Essential Facts

- Slipped capital femoral epiphysis is the most common hip abnormality to present in adolescence and early adulthood.
- The pain is usually described as a dull ache, exacerbated by activity.
- It is more common in males than females.
- It generally develops around the time of puberty.
- A Salter-Harris type I fracture occurs through the proximal femoral physis.
- Blood supply to the femoral epiphysis is through the femoral neck, so avascular necrosis develops in up to 20% of cases.
- A line drawn along the lateral aspect of the femoral neck should intersect the lateral aspect of the epiphysis.

✓ Pearls & ✗ Pitfalls

- ✓ The condition is associated with obesity.
- ✗ The contralateral hip is not always a safe basis for comparison because approximately 10% of patients have bilateral disease at presentation.

Case 92

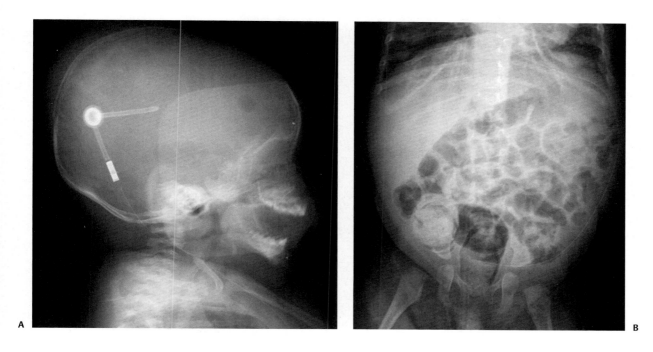

A B

■ Clinical Presentation

Lethargy in a 6-month-old with a history of ventriculoperitoneal shunt placement.

■ Imaging Findings

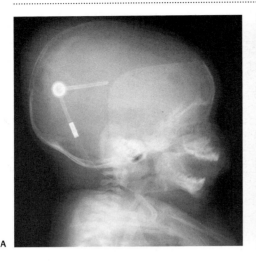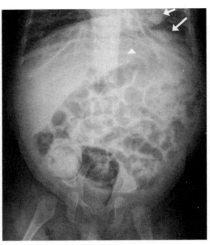

A   B

(A) A lateral radiograph of the skull demonstrates no disruption of the shunt catheter. **(B)** An abdominal radiograph obtained as part of the shunt series demonstrates the tip of the shunt catheter in the pelvis, with no evidence of disruption. However, there are bilateral rib fractures of varying ages, both old (with ample callus, *arrows*) and new (without evidence of healing, *arrowhead*).

■ Differential Diagnosis

- *Child abuse:* Except in rare settings of an underlying disease such as osteogenesis imperfecta or multiple episodes of accidental trauma, fractures of varying ages are essentially diagnostic of child abuse.
- *Osteogenesis imperfecta:* This is a rare condition associated with such radiographic findings as osteopenia and wormian bones (intrasutural ossifications).
- *Birth trauma:* Rib fractures rarely result from birth trauma and would have healed long before the child reached 6 months of age.

■ Essential Facts

- Child abuse accounts for approximately 1200 deaths per year in the United States.
- Fractures caused by abuse are most common before 3 years of age and account for 85% of child abuse fractures; of these, 50% occur within the first year of life.
- Fractures that are highly specific for intentional injury include classic metaphyseal lesions (metaphyseal corner fractures and bucket handle fractures); posterior rib fractures; fractures of the sternum, scapula, or spinous processes; and multiple fractures in various stages of healing.

■ Other Imaging Findings

- The American College of Radiology and the American Academy of Pediatrics highly recommend a skeletal survey if abuse is suspected.
- A full skeletal survey includes frontal and lateral views of the skull, chest, spine, upper arms and legs, and lower arms and legs; oblique views of the ribs; frontal and oblique views of both hands and feet; and a frontal view of the pelvis. The total number of images is approximately 31.
- In some situations, such as when abuse is strongly suspected, a follow-up skeletal survey should be obtained in 2 weeks.
- Fracture dating: Early fractures have soft-tissue obscuration secondary to hemorrhage and inflammation, with periosteal reaction usually apparent 4 to 14 days after the injury. Soft callus appears approximately 2 to 3 weeks after an injury, with hard callus at 3 to 6 weeks.
- Bone scan is a second-line supplement to the skeletal survey, providing a survey of the whole skeleton, although fractures of the skull and those near growth plates may be difficult to detect. Moreover, it does not permit dating of fractures.

✓ Pearls & ✗ Pitfalls

- ✓ Radiologists may be the first health professionals to detect signs of unsuspected child abuse on images obtained for other reasons.
- ✗ One of the most common reasons for missing the diagnosis of child abuse is the failure to consider it.

Case 93

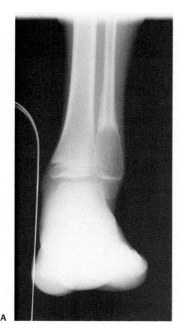

A

Clinical Presentation

A 7-year-old girl with pain and swelling in the left ankle and a limp for 2 to 3 months.

Further Work-up

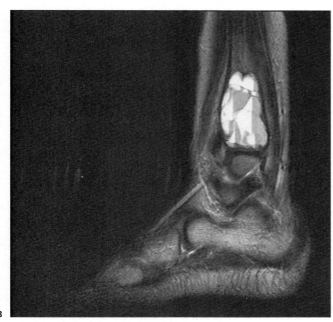

B

■ **Imaging Findings**

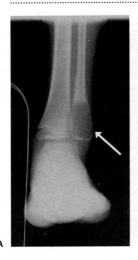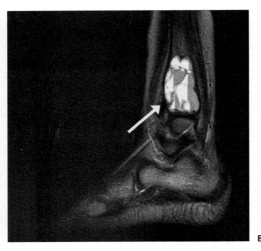

A   B

(A) Anteroposterior radiograph: There is a well-defined, expansile, lytic lesion in the metaphysis of the fibula with fine trabeculation (*arrow*). There is periosteal reaction. **(B)** Sagittal T2 image: There is an expansile, lobulated, septate lesion with a thin, well-defined rim of low signal intensity (*arrow*). There are fluid-fluid levels.

■ **Differential Diagnosis**

- ***Aneurysmal bone cyst (ABC):*** This lesion is characteristic of an ABC.
- *Solitary bone cyst:* This is always central in location, with little or no expansion, and less likely to contain fluid-fluid levels.
- *Telangiectatic osteosarcoma:* Also contains fluid-fluid levels, but usually has more bony destruction and lacks periosteal bone production. Can have an associated soft-tissue mass.

■ **Essential Facts**

- ABC rarely occurs in patients older than 30 years of age.
- It presents with rapidly increasing pain over 6 to 12 weeks.
- Can be primary or secondary. The secondary type occurs in conjunction with other lesions (chondroblastoma, non-ossifying fibroma, osteoblastoma, giant cell tumor, fibrous dysplasia, or a malignant tumor) or trauma.
- ABCs are treated with curettage and bone grafting; 20% recur after grafting.
- Plain radiographs: ABCs appear as "blowout" or "soap bubble" lesions that must be expansile.

■ **Other Imaging Findings**

- This is an expansile, non-neoplastic lytic lesion containing thin-walled, blood-filled cystic cavities. The cortex should be maintained. It is typically eccentric in location.
- ABC is most common in the metaphyses of long bones and posterior elements of the spine.
- Computed tomography and magnetic resonance imaging: Fluid-fluid levels are characteristic. The cyst contents do not enhance, but the septa will.
- Bone scan: There is a nonspecific accumulation of radioactive tracer at the periphery of the lesion, with less activity in the center.

✓ **Pearls & ✗ Pitfalls**

✓ ABC is rare in patients younger than 5 or older than 30 years.

✗ Fluid-fluid levels are characteristic of, but not pathognomonic for, ABC. They also occur in other lesions, including telangiectatic osteosarcoma.

✗ The differentiation of telangiectatic osteosarcoma and ABC can be difficult, but greater bony destruction is seen with telangiectatic osteosarcoma.

Case 94

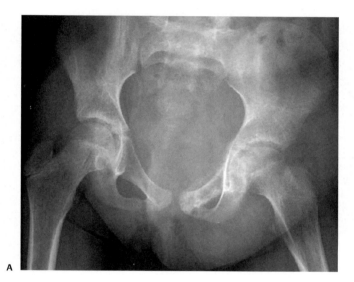

A

■ Clinical Presentation

A 9-year-old with progressive hip pain.

Further Work-up

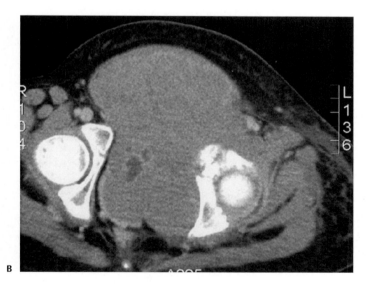

B

■ Imaging Findings

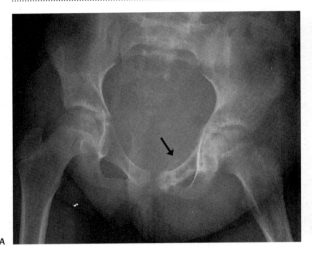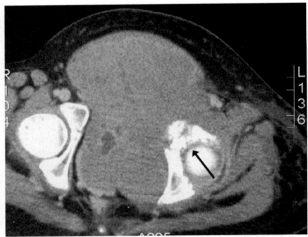

A   B

(A) Anteroposterior radiograph of the pelvis: there is an aggressive lesion in the left superior pubic ramus with a periosteal reaction (*arrow*) and an associated soft-tissue mass. **(B)** Axial computed tomography (CT) image: there is destruction of the left acetabulum (*arrow*), with an associated large soft-tissue mass.

■ Differential Diagnosis

- ***Ewing sarcoma:*** These findings are typical of Ewing sarcoma.
- *Osteosarcoma (OS):* Typically presents as a large, mixed sclerotic/lytic lesion with a cloudlike matrix. It is less likely to occur in flat bones.
- *Chondrosarcoma:* Most commonly occurs in patients older than 40 years and rarely in children.

■ Essential Facts

- Ewing sarcoma is a malignant tumor derived from undifferentiated mesenchymal cells of the bone marrow or primitive neuroectodermal cells (small, round, blue cell tumor).
- Age at presentation is 5 to 25 years. Peak age is 15 years. Ewing sarcoma is most common in white men, rare in African Americans.
- Signs and symptoms include localized pain and a soft-tissue mass with fever and leukocytosis.
- The presence of metastases (usually in the lung, but also the lymph nodes and other bones) is the best prognosticator.
- The 5-year survival rate of patients with locally resectable disease treated with chemotherapy is 75%. Patients with disseminated disease have a 5-year survival of 33%.
- This is an ill-defined intramedullary lesion with permeative bone destruction. The soft-tissue component tends to be disproportionately large compared with the bony destruction.
- Ewing sarcoma does not produce a tumor matrix.

- It can occur in any bone, but the diaphysis of a lower extremity is the most common location, followed by flat bones.
- Plain radiographic findings are as described above. May have an onion skin periosteal reaction, cortical erosion, sclerosis, thickening, and a noncalcified soft-tissue mass.
- Contrast CT shows heterogeneous enhancement.

■ Other Imaging Findings

- Magnetic resonance imaging (MRI): Typically has a low signal on T1 images and a high signal on T2 images.
- Bone scan demonstrates increased uptake of radioactive tracer.
- In addition to MRI of the primary tumor, bone scan and chest CT should be obtained to detect disseminated disease.
- Positron emission tomography can help assess the response to therapy.

✓ Pearls & ✗ Pitfalls

- ✓ It is sometimes difficult to differentiate Ewing sarcoma from OS. Ewing sarcoma is usually diaphyseal (OS is metaphyseal) and more common in the flat bones and axial skeleton. Ewing sarcoma has no tumor matrix (OS has a cloudlike matrix) and an onion skin periosteal reaction (OS has a sunburst appearance).
- ✗ Ewing sarcoma can look like and present identically to osteomyelitis.

Case 95

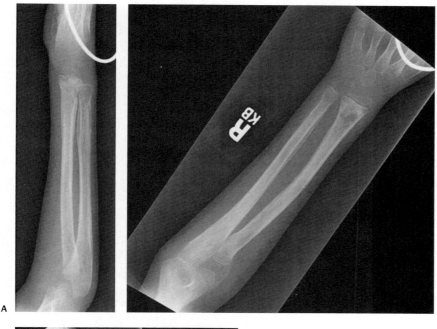

A

B

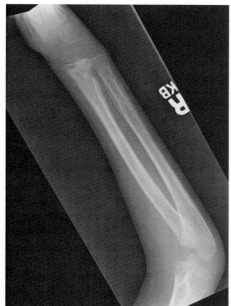

C

■ Clinical Presentation

An 8-year-old boy with fatigue and joint pain.

■ Imaging Findings

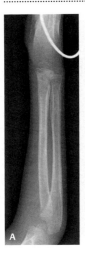 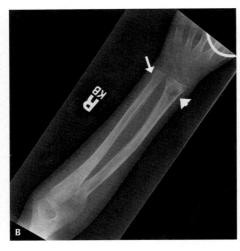 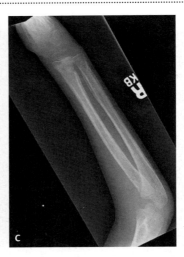

(A–C) Plain films: There is osteopenia, particularly in the carpal bones. In the distal ulna, there is a radiolucent transverse metaphyseal band with "moth-eaten" destruction of the proximal edge and a periosteal reaction (*arrow*). There is a focal osteolytic lesion in the distal radius (*arrowhead*).

■ Differential Diagnosis

- **Leukemia:** These films show multiple findings common in leukemia.
- *Osteomyelitis:* Can appear aggressive, similar to leukemia (periosteal reaction, bone destruction), and have similar symptoms. Transverse metaphyseal bands are more common in leukemia.
- *Metastatic neuroblastoma:* Often difficult to distinguish from leukemia. Can have metaphyseal bands and bone destruction.

■ Essential Facts

- Acute lymphocytic leukemia (ALL) is the most common leukemia of childhood. The peak age is 2 to 10 years, and boys are affected more often than girls.
- The most common signs and symptoms are recurrent joint pain, fatigue, fever, bleeding, hepatosplenomegaly, and adenopathy.
- Leukemia is treated with chemotherapy, radiation, granulocyte colony-stimulating factor, bone marrow transplant, and steroids.
- Complete remission is achieved in more than 90% of patients with ALL.
- In children, the most common bony location is the long bones (in adults, the axial skeleton).
- The disease can cause multiple flattened or biconcave vertebral bodies as well as horizontal leukemic lines.
- Chloroma (granulocytic sarcoma): This is a localized tumor consisting of immature colloid cells that is seen mainly in myeloid leukemia. The presence of a mass with destruction/production of bone in a patient with leukemia should suggest chloroma.

- Four types of bone changes have been traditionally described that generally resolve after therapy:
  - "Leukemic lines": transverse, radiolucent metaphyseal bands in large joints
  - Subperiosteal new bone formation along the shafts of long bones that can be smooth, lamellar, or sunburst in appearance
  - Focal destructive lesions
  - Diffuse sclerosis

■ Other Imaging Findings

- Bone scan shows increased uptake of radioactive tracer in involved areas.
- Magnetic resonance imaging (MRI)
  - T1: Hypointense signal replaces normal high signal in bone marrow.
  - T2/short inversion recovery: Increased signal is seen in the bone marrow.

✓ Pearls & ✗ Pitfalls

- ✓ Moth-eaten bony destruction and leukemic lines are characteristic.
- ✓ After therapy, there can be dense metaphyseal bands.
- ✓ MRI is often positive when the radiographs are negative.
- ✗ Bone scan may underestimate disease.

Case 96

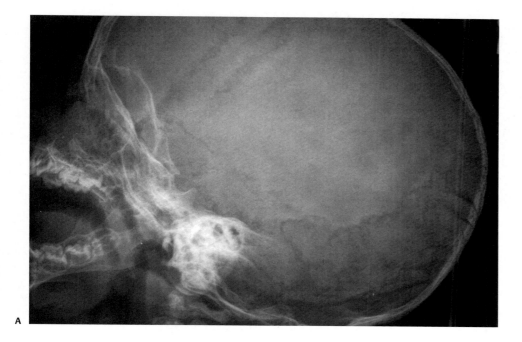

A

■ Clinical Presentation

A newborn with fractures.

Further Work-up

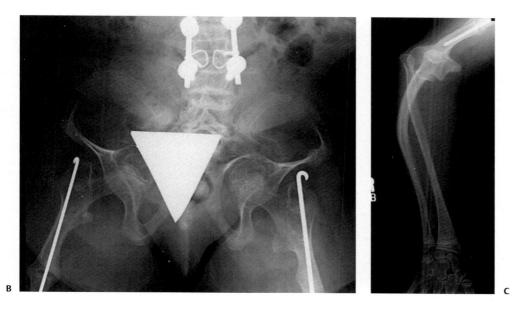

B

C

Later in life.

■ Imaging Findings

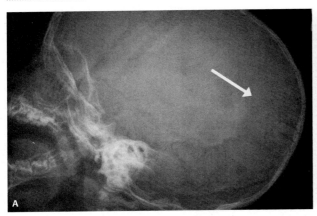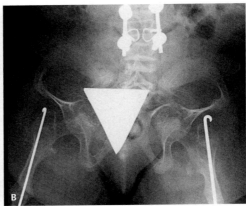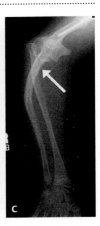

(A) Lateral view of the skull: there are multiple intrasutural (wormian) bones (*arrow*). **(B)** Anteroposterior view of the pelvis: There is severe protrusion of the acetabuli, coxa vara, and an old fracture of the right femur. The femora are thin and contain intramedullary rods. The lumbar vertebral bodies are biconcave and flattened. There are scoliosis rods. **(C)** Anteroposterior view of the forearm: There is bowing of the ulna (*arrow*) and a fracture of the distal humerus, which contains an intramedullary rod. There are thin, sclerotic metaphyseal bands parallel to the physis.

■ Differential Diagnosis

- ***Osteogenesis imperfecta (OI):*** All of the above findings are consistent with OI.
- *Rickets:* Can have intrasutural bones in the healing phase, protrusio acetabuli, coxa vara, and osteopenia. The wrist would demonstrate widened physes with cupped and frayed metaphyses.
- *Hypophosphatasia:* Involves osteopenia, multiple fractures, and intrasutural bones. Cranial synostosis may occur.

■ Essential Facts

- There are multiple types of OI, all of which have a type 1 collagen abnormality. OI varies in severity from mild (type 1) to lethal (type 2).
- Brainstem and cranial nerve compression can occur and lead to hearing loss.
- The face may appear triangular because of macrocranium and underdeveloped facial bones. Blue sclera, lax ligaments, and thin skin may also be apparent.
- The treatment includes bisphosphonates, physical therapy, and surgery to manage complications.
- Multiple fractures occur in thin, overtubulated bones.
- Skull: macrocranium with frontal bossing, wide sutures with intrasutural bones, basilar impression/invagination
- Spine: biconcave or flat vertebral bodies, spondylolisthesis
- Chest: sternal bowing and thoracic deformity
- Pelvis/hips: coxa vara and protrusio acetabuli
- Long bones: thin cortex, overtubulation and bowing, "popcorn" calcification in metaphyses (in certain types of OI), hyperplastic callus formation
- Feet: flatfoot and skew foot deformities

✓ Pearls & ✗ Pitfalls

- ✓ The differential diagnosis for intrasutural bones also includes the following: pyknodysostosis, rickets (healing), kinky hair syndrome, cleidocranial dysostosis, hypothyroidism/hypophosphatasia, otopalatodigital syndrome, primary acro-osteolysis (Hajdu-Cheney syndrome)/pachydermoperiostosis/progeria, Down syndrome.
- ✓ The thin metaphyseal bands parallel to the physis are due to cycles of bisphosphonate therapy.
- ✗ The various types of OI have varied radiographic features. It is not possible to type a case of OI strictly by the radiographic findings.

Case 97

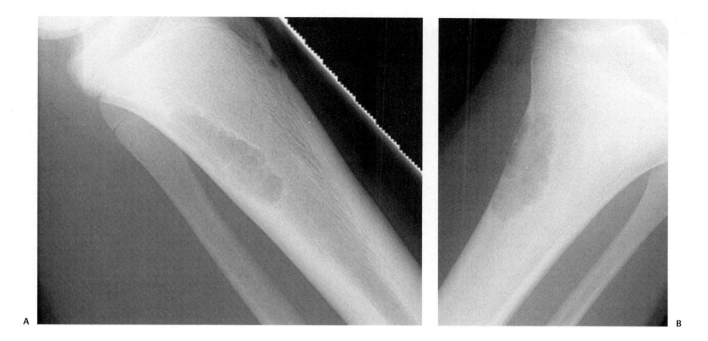

■ Clinical Presentation

A 16-year-old boy with pain after twisting his knee.

■ **Imaging Findings**

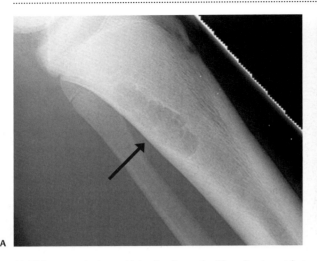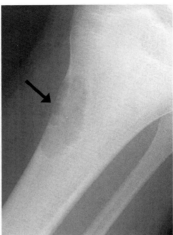

A   B

(A,B) Anteroposterior and lateral radiographs: There is a lucent lesion in the posteromedial cortex of the tibia with a thin, scalloped sclerotic border (*arrows*). There is no associated periostitis.

■ **Differential Diagnosis**

All three of the following lesions occur in patients who are younger than 30 years old.

- **Nonossifying fibroma (NOF):** A blister-like lesion in the cortex of the metaphysis of a long bone with a thin sclerotic border in a patient who is younger than 30 years old is most likely an NOF. There should be no periositis or pain (unless a pathologic fracture is present).
- *Aneurysmal bone cyst:* Should be more expansile and may have periostitis. The patient typically presents because of pain.
- *Solitary bone cyst:* Should be central in location rather than cortically based.

■ **Essential Facts**

- NOF is the most common fibrous lesion of bone, occurring in up to 20% of children.
- It is also called *fibrous cortical defect* (although some authors suggest that fibrous cortical defects are < 2 cm, whereas NOFs are > 2 cm).
- This is a benign lesion, and no action is needed.
- NOF appears as a well-defined, eccentric, lytic lesion with scalloped or smooth sclerotic margins in the intact cortex of the metaphysis of a long bone.
- There is no internal matrix.
- NOF usually appears as a single lesion about the knee in the posteromedial cortex. It is uncommon in the upper extremities.

- The lesion is usually metaphyseal, arising close to the growth plate, but with growth of the bone it can extend into the diaphysis.
- Sclerosis routinely develops over 2 to 4 years, and the NOF eventually disappears.

■ **Other Imaging Findings**

- Imaging methods other than plain films are not usually required because of the specificity of the radiographic findings.
- NOF demonstrates contrast enhancement.

✓ **Pearls & ✗ Pitfalls**

- ✓ The patient must be younger than 30 years old.
- ✓ There must be no associated periositis or pain (unless a pathologic fracture is present).
- ✓ The lesion must be cortically based.
- ✗ If computed tomography or magnetic resonance image is obtained, interruption of the cortex may be demonstrated. This must not be mistaken for cortical destruction.

Case 98

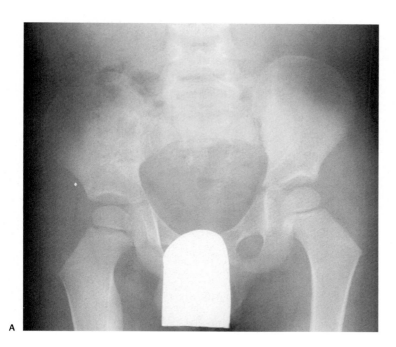

A

■ Clinical Presentation

A 6-year-old boy with hip pain.

Further Work-up

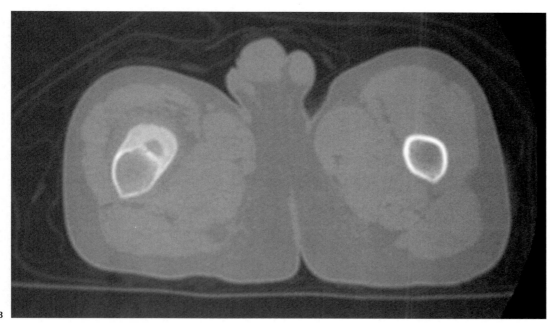

B

■ Imaging Findings

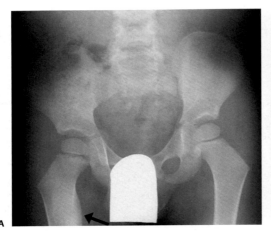
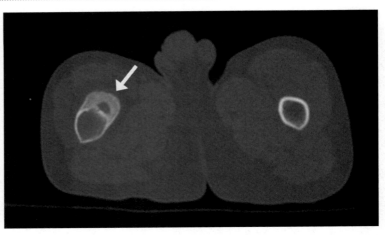

A B

(A) Anteroposterior radiograph of the pelvis: there is sclerosis of the proximal diaphysis of the right femur that is incompletely imaged (*arrow*). **(B)** Axial computed tomography (CT) image: there is a central, well-defined lytic lesion with thick subperiosteal new bone formation (*arrow*).

■ Differential Diagnosis

- ***Osteoid osteoma:*** These findings are consistent with osteoid osteoma.
- *Osteomyelitis (Brodie abscess):* This can be difficult to differentiate from osteoid osteoma. Often, there is a lucent tract extending from the nidus, as well as cortical destruction.
- *Stress fracture:* This can have surrounding sclerosis, but the central lucency is usually more linear and perpendicular to the cortex.

■ Essential Facts

- Osteoid osteoma is a benign tumor of unknown etiology consisting of an osteoblastic mass (nidus) smaller than 2 cm surrounded by reactive sclerosis.
- Patients are most commonly 10 to 25 years of age; the condition is two to three times more common in males.
- Signs and symptoms include local pain that is worse at night and exacerbated by alcohol. The pain is markedly relieved by aspirin.
- The lesion can regress spontaneously.
- Treatment: Surgical resection of the nidus, percutaneous radio-frequency ablation, or thermocoagulation is curative.
- The lesion can recur if the nidus is not completely removed.
- A well-defined lytic or sclerotic nidus is surrounded by exuberant sclerosis.
- Osteoid osteoma most commonly occurs in the metaphysis or diaphysis of long bones (usually the femur or tibia) but can occur in the phalanges and spine. It is rare in the skull.
- In cancellous or intra-articular lesions, there may be only mild reactive sclerosis with distant periostitis.

■ Other Imaging Findings

- Magnetic resonance imaging
  - T1: Nidus is isointense to muscle.
  - T2: Nidus shows intermediate to high signal. Peak contrast enhancement occurs during the arterial phase with early partial washout. Extensive bone marrow edema may be present, which can obscure the nidus.
- Bone scan: Uptake of radioactive tracer is increased. May appear as a small focus of intense activity surrounded by a larger area of increased activity.
- Angiography: Vascularity is increased in the region of the lesion with dense enhancement of the nidus. A feeding vessel may be identified.

✓ Pearls & ✗ Pitfalls

- ✓ Identifying the nidus is key. CT is the study of choice.
- ✓ In a patient with painful scoliosis, the lesion is located on the concave side.
- ✗ An osteoblastoma has an appearance similar to that of an osteoid osteoma, but the nidus is larger than 2 cm.

Case 99

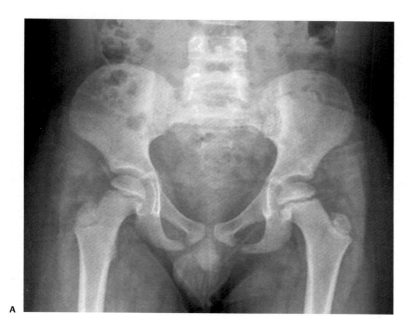

A

■ Clinical Presentation

A 5-year-old with a limp.

Further Work-up

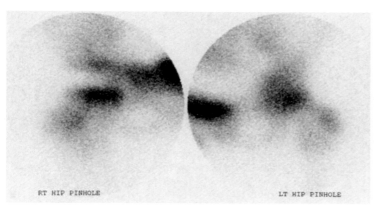

B

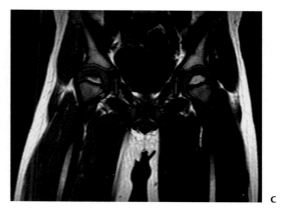

C

■ Imaging Findings

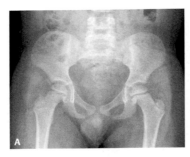
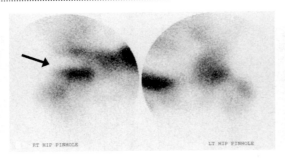
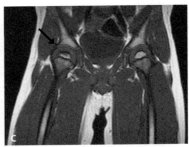

(A) Plain film: Both hips appear normal. There is no sclerosis, flattening, or fragmentation. **(B)** Nuclear medicine methylene diphosphonate (MDP) bone scan of both hips: On the pinhole views, there is decreased activity in the right femoral head (*arrow*). **(C)** Magnetic resonance imaging (MRI): T1 shows a hypointense, irregular area in the periphery of the right femoral head (*arrow*).

■ Differential Diagnosis

- **Legg-Calvé-Perthes disease (avascular necrosis [AVN]):** In early Perthes disease, a decrease in the blood supply to the epiphysis causes a cold defect on the bone scan that may not yet be evident on plain film. A hypointense area along the periphery of the epiphysis is also consistent with AVN.
- *Juvenile chronic arthritis:* This causes epiphyseal erosions that can appear similar to the MRI findings, but it also causes joint effusions and synovial hypertrophy, which are not seen. On bone scan, it usually demonstrates increased blood flow and radiotracer around the joints.
- *Toxic synovitis:* Can cause a significant effusion to explain the MDP scan findings, but the bone would appear normal on MRI.

■ Essential Facts

- AVN is caused by insufficiency of the capital epiphyseal blood supply, which leads to infarctions, trabecular fracture, and loss of height.
- Fifteen to 20% of cases are bilateral.
- The most common presenting sign/symptom is a limp with decreased range of motion in a patient without a history of trauma.
- The typical age is 3 to 10 years; AVN is four times more common in boys.
- The younger the patient at presentation, the better the prognosis.
- Treatment is conservative; 50% of patients improve without treatment. Femoral or pelvic osteotomies can help to contain the hip.
- AVN can lead to a discrepancy in leg length and atrophy of the thigh.

■ Other Imaging Findings

- Plain film: The earliest change is mild lateral displacement of the femoral head due to joint effusion. Sclerosis, fragmentation, and flattening of the epiphysis occur later. Subchondral lucency indicates fracture. Later findings include coxa plana and coxa magna.
- MRI: T1 and T2 show hypointense irregularity along the periphery of the ossification center. As revascularization occurs, the hypointensity becomes replaced with bone marrow fat signal.
- Nuclear medicine: Changes occur earlier than radiographic changes. Early decreased uptake is followed by increased uptake as revascularization occurs.

✓ Pearls & ✗ Pitfalls

- ✓ The typical patient is a thin, 6-year-old boy.
- ✓ MRI is most sensitive in detecting early changes.

Case 100

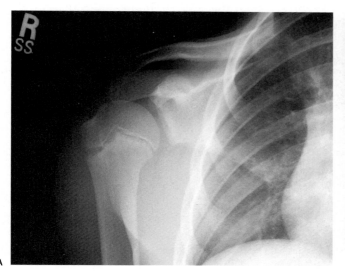

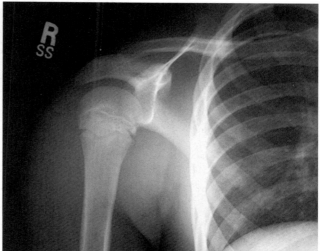

■ Clinical Presentation

A 12-year-old with right shoulder pain after trauma.

Further Work-up

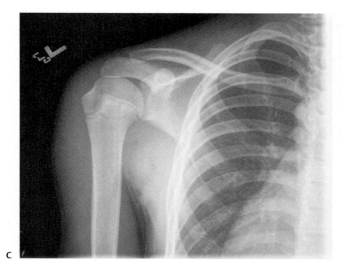

Reversed left shoulder radiograph for comparison.

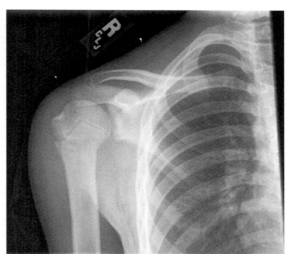

Right shoulder 1 week later.

■ Imaging Findings

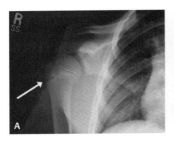
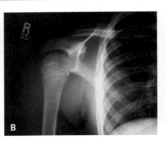
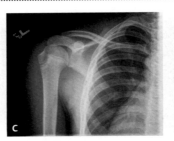
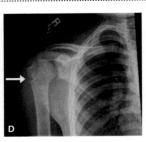

(A,B) Anteroposterior radiographs of the right shoulder: There is subtle widening of the growth plate laterally (*arrow*). It is not apparent on the internal rotation film. **(C)** Anteroposterior radiograph of the left shoulder: the growth plate is more uniform in appearance. **(D)** Anteroposterior radiograph of the right shoulder 1 week later: there is now a periosteal reaction, confirming the fracture (*arrow*).

■ Differential Diagnosis

- *Salter-Harris type I fracture:* The subtle widening of the growth plate, which is asymmetric in comparison with the contralateral one, is consistent with fracture.
- *Normal shoulder:* Subsequent periosteal reaction rules this out.
- *Other types of Salter-Harris fracture:* Only widening of the growth plate is identified. A careful search for a fracture line through the epiphysis or metaphysis rules this out.

■ Essential Facts

- In children, the joint capsule and ligaments are stronger than the physis, so that disruption of the physis occurs before damage to the ligaments and joint capsule.
- There are at least nine different types of Salter-Harris fractures, but types I through V are the most common:
  - Type I: fracture through the physis only (5%)
  - Type II: fracture through physis and metaphysis (75%)
  - Type III: fracture through physis and epiphysis (5%)
  - Type IV: fracture through physis, epiphysis, and metaphysis (10%)
  - Type V: crush fracture involving the physis (rare)
- Treatment includes casting for the lower categories, open reduction and internal fixation for the higher categories.
- Complications include premature epiphyseal closure leading to limb shortening or joint angulation.

■ Other Imaging Findings

- Computed tomography: may be helpful to evaluate extent of the fracture and degree of displacement of the physis.
- Magnetic resonance imaging: may be helpful to detect premature closure of the physis or occult fractures.
  - T1: fracture will appear as a low-signal line.
  - T2: increased signal is identified in bone marrow and surrounding soft tissue.

✓ Pearls & ✗ Pitfalls

- ✓ If a Salter-Harris type I fracture is suspected, contralateral radiographs may be helpful for comparison.
- ✗ Salter-Harris type I fractures can be difficult to identify. If they are suspected but not identified, follow-up radiographs in 7 to 10 days may be helpful to show healing.

Further Readings

Case 1

Keckler SJ, St Peter SD, Valusek PA, et al. VACTERL anomalies in patients with esophageal atresia: an updated delineation of the spectrum and review of the literature. Pediatr Surg Int 2007;23(4):309–313

Case 2

Siu CW, Cheung SC, Chan CW, Lam YM, Tse HF, Jim MH. Scimitar syndrome on chest x ray. Postgrad Med J 2008;84(996):558

Woodring JH, Howard TA, Kanga JF. Congenital pulmonary venolobar syndrome revisited. Radiographics 1994;14(2):349–369

Case 3

Farrugia MK, Raza SA, Gould S, Lakhoo K. Congenital lung lesions: classification and concordance of radiological appearance and surgical pathology. Pediatr Surg Int 2008;24(9):987–991

Johnson AM, Hubbard AM. Congenital anomalies of the fetal/neonatal chest. Semin Roentgenol 2004;39(2):197–214

Case 4

Crowley JJ, Sarnaik S. Imaging of sickle cell disease. Pediatr Radiol 1999;29(9):646–661

Kumar DS, Yadavali RP, Concepcion LA, Aniq H. Acute chest pain in a young woman with a chronic illness. Br J Radiol 2008;81(963):261–263

Case 5

Cleveland RH. A radiologic update on medical diseases of the newborn chest. Pediatr Radiol 1995;25(8):631–637

Hermansen CL, Lorah KN. Respiratory distress in the newborn. Am Fam Physician 2007;76(7):987–994

Case 6

Kransdorf MJ, Bancroft LW, Peterson JJ, Murphey MD, Foster WC, Temple HT. Imaging of fatty tumors: distinction of lipoma and well-differentiated liposarcoma. Radiology 2002;224(1):99–104

Case 7

Mehta K, Haller JO, Legasto AC. Imaging neuroblastoma in children. Crit Rev Computed Tomogr 2003;44(1):47–61

Case 8

Waag KL, Loff S, Zahn K, et al. Congenital diaphragmatic hernia: a modern day approach. Semin Pediatr Surg 2008;17(4):244–254

Case 9

Sobol SE, Zapata S. Epiglottitis and croup. Otolaryngol Clin North Am 2008;41(3):551–566, ix

Case 10

Griesdale DE, Bosma TL, Kurth T, Isac G, Chittock DR. Complications of endotracheal intubation in the critically ill. Intensive Care Med 2008;34(10):1835–1842

Case 11

Shah S, Sharieff GQ. Pediatric respiratory infections. Emerg Med Clin North Am 2007;25(4):961–979, vi

Case 12

Feja K, Saiman L. Tuberculosis in children. Clin Chest Med 2005;26(2):295–312, vii

Case 13

Fitzgerald DA. Congenital cyst adenomatoid malformations: resect some and observe all? Paediatr Respir Rev 2007;8(1):67–76

Case 14

Apostolopoulou SC, Kelekis NL, Brountzos EN, Rammos S, Kelekis DA. "Absent" pulmonary artery in one adult and five pediatric patients: imaging, embryology, and therapeutic implications. AJR Am J Roentgenol 2002;179(5):1253–1260

Case 15

Lozano JM. Bronchiolitis. Clin Evid 2005;14(14):285–297

Case 16

Shi HS, Yang F, Han P, et al. Findings of chest radiograph and spiral computed tomography in Swyer-James syndrome. Chin Med Sci J 2006;21(1):53–56

Case 17

Hernanz-Schulman M. Vascular rings: a practical approach to imaging diagnosis. Pediatr Radiol 2005;35(10):961–979

Case 18

Jassal MS, Benson JE, Mogayzel PJ Jr. Spontaneous resolution of diffuse persistent pulmonary interstitial emphysema. Pediatr Pulmonol 2008;43(6):615–619

Johnson AM, Hubbard AM. Congenital anomalies of the fetal/neonatal chest. Semin Roentgenol 2004;39(2):197–214

Case 19

Castañer E, Gallardo X, Rimola J, et al. Congenital and acquired pulmonary artery anomalies in the adult: radiologic overview. Radiographics 2006;26(2):349–371

Case 20

Ferguson EC, Krishnamurthy R, Oldham SA. Classic imaging signs of congenital cardiovascular abnormalities. Radiographics 2007;27(5):1323–1334

Case 21

Paranon S, Acar P. Ebstein's anomaly of the tricuspid valve: from fetus to adult: congenital heart disease. Heart 2008;94(2):237–243

Case 22

Duong M, Wenger J. Lemierre syndrome. Pediatr Emerg Care 2005;21(9):589–593

Case 23

McAdams HP, Kirejczyk WM, Rosado-de-Christenson ML, Matsumoto S. Bronchogenic cyst: imaging features with clinical and histopathologic correlation. Radiology 2000;217(2):441–446

Case 24

Kramer SS, Wehunt WD, Stocker JT, Kashima H. Pulmonary manifestations of juvenile laryngotracheal papillomatosis. AJR Am J Roentgenol 1985;144(4):687–694

Case 25

Wood BP. Cystic fibrosis: 1997. Radiology 1997;204(1):1–10

Case 26

Cheng G, Soboleski D, Daneman A, Poenaru D, Hurlbut D. Sonographic pitfalls in the diagnosis of enteric duplication cysts. AJR Am J Roentgenol 2005;184(2):521–525

Case 27

Roos JE, Pfiffner R, Stallmach T, Stuckmann G, Marincek B, Willi U. Infantile hemangioendothelioma. Radiographics 2003;23(6):1649–1655
van der Meijs BB, Merks JH, de Haan TR, Tabbers MM, van Rijn RR. Neonatal hepatic haemangioendothelioma: treatment options and dilemmas. Pediatr Radiol 2009;39(3):277–281

Case 28

Diamond IR, Casadiego G, Traubici J, Langer JC, Wales PW. The contrast enema for Hirschsprung disease: predictors of a false-positive result. J Pediatr Surg 2007;42(5):792–795

Case 29

Gupta AK, Guglani B. Imaging of congenital anomalies of the gastrointestinal tract. Indian J Pediatr 2005;72(5):403–414

Case 30

Perks AE, MacNeily AE, Blair GK. Posterior urethral valves. J Pediatr Surg 2002;37(7):1105–1107

Case 31

Sutherland DE, Jarrett TW. Surgical options in the management of ureteropelvic junction obstruction. Curr Urol Rep 2009;10(1):23–28

Case 32

Thurley PD, Halliday KE, Somers JM, Al-Daraji WI, Ilyas M, Broderick NJ. Radiological features of Meckel's diverticulum and its complications. Clin Radiol 2009;64(2):109–118

Case 33

Hernanz-Schulman M. Infantile hypertrophic pyloric stenosis. Radiology 2003;227(2):319–331

Case 34

Siegel MJ. Pelvic tumors in childhood. Radiol Clin North Am 1997;35(6):1455–1475
Tateishi U, Hosono A, Makimoto A, et al. Comparative study of FDG PET/CT and conventional imaging in the staging of rhabdomyosarcoma. Ann Nucl Med 2009;23(2):155–161

Case 35

Wootton-Gorges SL, Thomas KB, Harned RK, Wu SR, Stein-Wexler R, Strain JD. Giant cystic abdominal masses in children. Pediatr Radiol 2005;35(12):1277–1288

Case 36

Buonomo C. Neonatal gastrointestinal emergencies. Radiol Clin North Am 1997;35(4):845–864

Case 37

Delaney L, Applegate KE, Karmazyn B, Akisik MF, Jennings SG. MR cholangiopancreatography in children: feasibility, safety, and initial experience. Pediatr Radiol 2008;38(1):64–75

Case 38

Traubici J. The double bubble sign. Radiology 2001;220(2):463–464 PubMed

Case 39

Aspelund G, Langer JC. Current management of hypertrophic pyloric stenosis. Semin Pediatr Surg 2007;16(1):27–33

Case 40

Hajivassiliou CA. Intestinal obstruction in neonatal/pediatric surgery. Semin Pediatr Surg 2003;12(4):241–253

Case 41

Sizemore AW, Rabbani KZ, Ladd A, Applegate KE. Diagnostic performance of the upper gastrointestinal series in the evaluation of children with clinically suspected malrotation. Pediatr Radiol 2008;38(5):518–528

Case 42

Guner YS, Chokshi N, Petrosyan M, Upperman JS, Ford HR, Grikscheit TC. Necrotizing enterocolitis—bench to bedside: novel and emerging strategies. Semin Pediatr Surg 2008;17(4):255–265

Case 43

Bundy DG, Byerley JS, Liles EA, Perrin EM, Katznelson J, Rice HE. Does this child have appendicitis? JAMA 2007;298(4):438–451

Case 44

Schreuder MF, Westland R, van Wijk JA. Unilateral multicystic dysplastic kidney: a meta-analysis of observational studies on the incidence, associated urinary tract malformations and the contralateral kidney. Nephrol Dial Transplant 2009;24(6):1810–1818

Case 45

Grattan-Smith JD, Blews DE, Brand T. Omental infarction in pediatric patients: sonographic and CT findings. AJR Am J Roentgenol 2002;178(6):1537–1539

Case 46

Hopkins JK, Giles HW Jr, Wyatt-Ashmead J, Bigler SA. Best cases from the AFIP: cystic nephroma. Radiographics 2004;24(2):589–593

Case 47

Lowe LH, Isuani BH, Heller RM, et al. Pediatric renal masses: Wilms tumor and beyond. Radiographics 2000;20(6):1585–1603

Case 48

Ko HS, Schenk JP, Tröger J, Rohrschneider WK. Current radiological management of intussusception in children. Eur Radiol 2007;17(9):2411–2421

Case 49

Miltenburg DM, Schaffer R III, Breslin T, Brandt ML. Changing indications for pediatric cholecystectomy. Pediatrics 2000;105(6):1250–1253

Case 50

Lowe ME, Greer JB. Pancreatitis in children and adolescents. Curr Gastroenterol Rep 2008;10(2):128–135

Case 51

Brisse HJ, Smets AM, Kaste SC, Owens CM. Imaging in unilateral Wilms tumour. Pediatr Radiol 2008;38(1):18–29

Case 52

Roebuck DJ, Olsen O, Pariente D. Radiological staging in children with hepatoblastoma. Pediatr Radiol 2006;36(3):176–182

Case 53

Lynch KA, Feola PG, Guenther E. Gastric trichobezoar: an important cause of abdominal pain presenting to the pediatric emergency department. Pediatr Emerg Care 2003;19(5):343–347

Case 54

Shokeir AA, Nijman RJ. Ureterocele: an ongoing challenge in infancy and childhood. BJU Int 2002;90(8):777–783

Case 55

Dogan HS, Tekgul S. Management of pediatric stone disease. Curr Urol Rep 2007;8(2):163–173

Case 56

Johnson S, Taylor CM. What's new in haemolytic uraemic syndrome? Eur J Pediatr 2008;167(9):965–971

Case 57

Smith EA. Pyelonephritis, renal scarring, and reflux nephropathy: a pediatric urologist's perspective. Pediatr Radiol 2008;38(Suppl 1):S76–S82

Case 58

Bauer R, Kogan BA. New developments in the diagnosis and management of pediatric UTIs. Urol Clin North Am 2008;35(1):47–58, vi

Case 59

Torres VE, Harris PC. Mechanisms of disease: autosomal dominant and recessive polycystic kidney diseases. Nat Clin Pract Nephrol 2006;2(1):40–55, quiz 55

Case 60

Grantham JJ. Clinical practice. Autosomal dominant polycystic kidney disease. N Engl J Med 2008;359(14):1477–1485

Case 61

Blei F. Congenital lymphatic malformations. Ann N Y Acad Sci 2008; 1131:185–194

Case 62

Sala E. Magnetic resonance imaging of the female pelvis. Semin Roentgenol 2008;43(4):290–302

Case 63

Lin EP, Bhatt S, Rubens DJ, Dogra VS. Testicular torsion: twists and turns. Semin Ultrasound CT MR 2007;28(4):317–328

Case 64

Kamaya A, Shin L, Chen B, Desser TS. Emergency gynecologic imaging. Semin Ultrasound CT MR 2008;29(5):353–368

Case 65

de Silva KS, Kanumakala S, Grover SR, Chow CW, Warne GL. Ovarian lesions in children and adolescents—an 11-year review. J Pediatr Endocrinol Metab 2004;17(7):951–957

Case 66

Westra SJ, Zaninovic AC, Hall TR, Kangarloo H, Boechat MI. Imaging of the adrenal gland in children. Radiographics 1994;14(6):1323–1340

Case 67

Provenzale J. CT and MR imaging of acute cranial trauma. Emerg Radiol 2007;14(1):1–12

Case 68

Koeller KK, Sandberg GD; Armed Forces Institute of Pathology. From the archives of the AFIP. Cerebral intraventricular neoplasms: radiologic-pathologic correlation. Radiographics 2002;22(6):1473–1505

Case 69

Robbin MR, Murphey MD, Temple HT, Kransdorf MJ, Choi JJ. Imaging of musculoskeletal fibromatosis. Radiographics 2001;21(3):585–600

Case 70

Christophe C, Bartholome J, Blum D, et al. Neonatal tuberous sclerosis. US, CT, and MR diagnosis of brain and cardiac lesions. Pediatr Radiol 1989;19(6-7):446–448
Plensdorf S, Martinez J. Common pigmentation disorders. Am Fam Physician 2009;79(2):109–116

Case 71

Arekapudi SR, Varma DR. Lingual thyroid. Pediatr Radiol 2007; 37(9):940

Case 72

Koeller KK, Rushing EJ. From the archives of the AFIP: medulloblastoma: a comprehensive review with radiologic-pathologic correlation. Radiographics 2003;23(6):1613–1637

Case 73

Eldevik OP, Blaivas M, Gabrielsen TO, Hald JK, Chandler WF. Craniopharyngioma: radiologic and histologic findings and recurrence. AJNR Am J Neuroradiol 1996;17(8):1427–1439

Case 74

Santaolalla F, Araluce I, Zabala A, López A, Garay M, Sanchez JM. Efficacy of selective percutaneous embolization for the treatment of intractable posterior epistaxis and juvenile nasopharyngeal angiofibroma (JNA). Acta Otolaryngol 2009;129(12):1456–1462

Case 75

Hahn JS, Lewis AJ, Barnes P. Hydranencephaly owing to twin-twin transfusion: serial fetal ultrasonography and magnetic resonance imaging findings. J Child Neurol 2003;18(5):367–370

Case 76

Phelan JA, Lowe LH, Glasier CM. Pediatric neurodegenerative white matter processes: leukodystrophies and beyond. Pediatr Radiol 2008;38(7):729–749

Case 77

Hayashi N, Tsutsumi Y, Barkovich AJ. Morphological features and associated anomalies of schizencephaly in the clinical population: detailed analysis of MR images. Neuroradiology 2002;44(5):418–427

Case 78

Alvarez H, Garcia Monaco R, Rodesch G, Sachet M, Krings T, Lasjaunias P. Vein of Galen aneurysmal malformations. Neuroimaging Clin N Am 2007;17(2):189–206

Case 79

Naradzay JF, Browne BJ, Rolnick MA, Doherty RJ. Cerebral ventricular shunts. J Emerg Med 1999;17(2):311–322

Case 80

Richer LP, Sinclair DB, Bhargava R. Neuroimaging features of acute disseminated encephalomyelitis in childhood. Pediatr Neurol 2005;32(1):30–36

Case 81

Lemyre E, Azouz EM, Teebi AS, Glanc P, Chen MF. Bone dysplasia series. Achondroplasia, hypochondroplasia and thanatophoric dysplasia: review and update. Can Assoc Radiol J 1999;50(3):185–197

Case 82

Misra M, Pacaud D, Petryk A, Collett-Solberg PF, Kappy M; Drug and Therapeutics Committee of the Lawson Wilkins Pediatric Endocrine Society. Vitamin D deficiency in children and its management: review of current knowledge and recommendations. Pediatrics 2008;122(2):398–417

Case 83

Fernandez M, Carrol CL, Baker CJ. Discitis and vertebral osteomyelitis in children: an 18-year review. Pediatrics 2000;105(6):1299–1304

Case 84

Pahade J, Sekhar A, Shetty SK. Imaging of malignant skeletal tumors. Cancer Treat Res 2008;143:367–422

Case 85

Robbin MR, Murphey MD. Benign chondroid neoplasms of bone. Semin Musculoskelet Radiol 2000;4(1):45–58

Case 86

Jadhav SP, Swischuk LE. Commonly missed subtle skeletal injuries in children: a pictorial review. Emerg Radiol 2008;15(6):391–398

Case 87

Omid R, Choi PD, Skaggs DL. Supracondylar humeral fractures in children. J Bone Joint Surg Am 2008;90(5):1121–1132

Case 88

Young AJ, McAllister DR. Evaluation and treatment of tibial stress fractures. Clin Sports Med 2006;25(1):117–128, x

Case 89

Rossi F, Dragoni S. Acute avulsion fractures of the pelvis in adolescent competitive athletes: prevalence, location and sports distribution of 203 cases collected. Skeletal Radiol 2001;30(3):127–131

Case 90

DiGiovanni CW, Patel A, Calfee R, Nickisch F. Osteonecrosis in the foot. J Am Acad Orthop Surg 2007;15(4):208–217

Case 91

Aronsson DD, Loder RT, Breur GJ, Weinstein SL. Slipped capital femoral epiphysis: current concepts. J Am Acad Orthop Surg 2006;14(12):666–679

Case 92

Lonergan GJ, Baker AM, Morey MK, Boos SC. From the archives of the AFIP. Child abuse: radiologic-pathologic correlation. Radiographics 2003;23(4):811–845

Case 93

Mahnken AH, Nolte-Ernsting CC, Wildberger JE, et al. Aneurysmal bone cyst: value of MR imaging and conventional radiography. Eur Radiol 2003;13(5):1118–1124

Case 94

Iwamoto Y. Diagnosis and treatment of Ewing's sarcoma. Jpn J Clin Oncol 2007;37(2):79–89

Case 95

McKinstry CS, Steiner RE, Young AT, Jones L, Swirsky D, Aber V. Bone marrow in leukemia and aplastic anemia: MR imaging before, during, and after treatment. Radiology 1987;162(3):701–707

Case 96

Rauch F, Glorieux FH. Osteogenesis imperfecta. Lancet 2004;363 (9418):1377–1385

Case 97

Betsy M, Kupersmith LM, Springfield DS. Metaphyseal fibrous defects. J Am Acad Orthop Surg 2004;12(2):89–95

Case 98

Liu PT, Chivers FS, Roberts CC, Schultz CJ, Beauchamp CP. Imaging of osteoid osteoma with dynamic gadolinium-enhanced MR imaging. Radiology 2003;227(3):691–700

Case 99

Pasierbek M. Local experience in the diagnosis and treatment of Perthes' disease. Ortop Traumatol Rehabil 2001;3(3):354–356

Case 100

Swischuk LE, Hernandez JA. Frequently missed fractures in children (value of comparative views). Emerg Radiol 2004;11(1):22–28

Index

Note: Locators refer to case number. Locators in **boldface** indicate primary diagnosis.

A

Abscess
    abdominal, 61
    Brodie, 88, 98
    pelvic, 62
Achondroplasia, 81
Acute chest syndrome (ACS), in sickle cell disease, **4**
Acute disseminated encephalomyelitis (ADEM), **80**
Adenopathy, 7
Adrenal hemorrhage, **66**
Adrenoleukodystrophy, X-linked, **76**
Alobar holoprosencephaly, 75
Aneurysm, cerebral, true, 78
Aneurysmal bone cyst, **93**, 97
Angiomyolipoma, 6
Annular pancreas, 33
Anterior superior iliac spine, avulsion fracture, **89**
Aortic arch
    double, **17**
    right, with aberrant left subclavian artery, 17
Aortic coarctation. *See* Coarctation of
    aorta
Aortic stenosis, 20
Appendicitis, 32, **43**, 45, 48, 65
Arachnoid cyst, 73
Arthritis, 87
    of hip, 91
    juvenile chronic, 99
    septic, 86
Aspiration pneumonia, 4
Asthma, 15
Astrocytoma, pilocytic, 72
Avascular necrosis. *See also* Legg-Calvé-Perthes
    disease
    of capitellum, 87
Avulsion fracture, of anterior superior iliac spine,
    89

B

Bezoar, **53**
Biliary sludge, 49
Birth trauma, 92
Bladder
    extrinsic impression on, 54
    hematoma, 34
    mass in, 54
Blood clot, 55
Bone anatomy, normal, 58
Bone cyst
    aneurysmal, **93**, 97
    solitary, 93, 97

Bowel
    normal anatomy, 58
    obstruction, 42
        mechanical, **40**
BPD. *See* Bronchopulmonary dysplasia (BPD)
Branchial cleft abnormalities, 69
Brodie abscess, 88, 98
Bronchiolitis, viral, **15**
Bronchogenic cyst, 3, 11, **23**
Bronchopulmonary dysplasia (BPD), developing,
    18

C

Capitellum, avascular necrosis, 87
CBD. *See* Common bile duct
CCAM. *See* Congenital cystic adenomatous
    malformation
Cerebral aneurysm, true, 78
Cerebral contusion, 67
Cervical lymphadenopathy, 69
CF. *See* Cystic fibrosis
Child abuse, **92**
Choledochal cyst, **37**
Cholelithiasis, **49**
Chondroblastoma, **85**
Chondrosarcoma, 94
Choroid plexus carcinoma, **68**
Choroid plexus cyst, 78
Choroid plexus papilloma, **68**
CLE. *See* Congenital lobar emphysema
Coarctation of aorta, **20**
Coccidioidomycosis, 12
Common bile duct
    obstructing stone/mass, 37
    stricture, 37
Congenital adrenal hyperplasia, 66
Congenital cystic adenomatous malformation, 3
Congenital lobar emphysema, 16
Congenital pulmonary adenomatous malformation,
    8, **13**
Congenital pulmonary venolobar syndrome. *See*
    Scimitar syndrome
Contrast media, prior administration, versus
    vesicoureteral reflux, 58
CPAM. *See* Congenital pulmonary adenomatous
    malformation
CPCa. *See* Choroid plexus carcinoma
CPP. *See* Choroid plexus papilloma
Craniopharyngioma, **73**
Croup, 9
Cushing syndrome, 25

Cyst(s). *See also* Aneurysmal bone cyst; Esophageal
        duplication
    arachnoid, 73
    bronchogenic, 3, 11, **23**
    choledochal, **37**
    choroid plexus, 78
    duplication, **26**, 35
    mesenteric, 26
    ovarian, hemorrhagic, 64
    Rathke cleft, 73
    renal, simple, 60
    thyroglossal duct, 71
Cystic fibrosis, **25**
Cystic renal dysplasia, 59

D
Diaphragmatic hernia, congenital, **8**
Diskitis, **83**
Double aortic arch, **17**
Duodenal atresia, **38**
Duodenal obstruction, congenital, 41
Duodenal web, 33, 38
Duodenum, "wandering," 41
Duplication cyst, gastrointestinal, **26**, 35. *See also*
        Esophageal duplication

E
Ebstein anomaly (EA), **21**
Emphysema
    congenital lobar, 16
    pulmonary interstitial, **18**
Endotracheal tube
    bronchial intubation, 10
    esophageal intubation, **10**
    high position, 10
Ependymoma, 72
Epididymal appendage, torsion, 63
Epididymo-orchitis, 63
Epidural hematoma, **67**
Epiglottis
    normal variant, 9
    omega, 9
Epiglottitis, **9**
Epiploic appendagitis, 45
Esophageal duplication, 17, 23
Esophageal intubation, **10**
Esophageal perforation, 1
Esophageal tube
    esophageal perforation by, 1
    tracheal placement, 1
Ewing sarcoma, 84, **94**

F
Fibromatosis colli, **69**
Foregut malformation, 19. *See also* Bronchogenic
        cyst; Esophageal duplication
Fracture(s). *See also* Avulsion fracture; Child abuse

of hip
    acute, 89
    stress, 98
Salter-Harris, 100
    type 1, **100**
stress
    of hip, 98
    tibial, **88**
supracondylar, **87**
tibial, stress, **88**
toddler, **86**
Fungal disease, invasive, 24
Fungus ball, 55

G
Gallbladder polyp, 49
Ganglioneuroblastoma, 7
Ganglioneuroma, 7
Gastroesophageal reflux, 39
Gastrointestinal duplication cyst, **26**, 35
Gastroparesis, 53
Giant cell tumor, 85
Granulomatous disease, 12
Gray matter heterotopia, 70

H
Hemangioendotheliomatosis, **27**
Hematoma, 55
    epidural, **67**
    subdural, 67
Hematometrocolpos, 34
Hemolytic uremic syndrome, **56**
Henoch-Schönlein purpura, 56
Hepatoblastoma, 27, **52**
Hepatocellular carcinoma, 52
Hernia(s), hiatal, 13
Hiatal hernia, 13
Hip fracture
    acute, 89
    stress, 98
Hirschsprung disease, **28**
    total colonic, 36
Histoplasmosis, 12
Hydranencephaly, **75**
Hydrocephalus, severe, 75
Hydrometrocolpos, **62**
Hydronephrosis, 44
Hypersensitivity pneumonitis, 12
Hypertrophic pyloric stenosis, **33**, **39**
Hypogenetic lung syndrome, 14. *See also* Scimitar
        syndrome
Hypophosphatasia, 96

I
Ileal atresia, 29, **36**
Ileus, functional, 40, 42
Inflammatory bowel disease (IBD), 32

Intestinal duplication. *See also* Gastrointestinal
    duplication cyst
  containing gastric mucosa, 32
Intraventricular hemorrhage, 68
Intussusception, **48**

J
JNA. *See* Juvenile nasopharyngeal angiofibroma
Juvenile chronic arthritis, 99
Juvenile nasopharyngeal angiofibroma, **74**

K
Kidney. *See also* Polycystic kidney disease
    multicystic dysplastic, 31, **44**, 46
Kohler disease, **90**

L
Langerhans cell histiocytosis, spinal involvement, 83
Laryngotracheal papillomatosis, 22
Legg-Calvé-Perthes disease, 91, **99**
Lemierre syndrome, **22**
Leukemia(s), 47, 82, **95**
    spinal involvement, 83
Lingual thyroid, **71**
Lingual tonsil, enlarged, 71
Lipoma, **6**
Liposarcoma, 6
Liver, metastases to, 52
Lung(s). *See also* Pulmonary
    right, hypoplasia, 2, 14
Lymphadenopathy
    cervical, 69
    mediastinal, 19
    necrotic, 23
Lymphatic malformation, 26, **61**
Lymphoma(s), 47

M
Malrotation, with midgut volvulus, 38, 40, **41**
MCDK. *See* Multicystic dysplastic kidney
Meckel diverticulum, **32**, 43, 48
Meconium aspiration, **5**
Meconium ileus, 28, **29**, 36
Meconium plug, 28
Meconium plug syndrome, 29
Meconium pseudocyst, **35**
Medulloblastoma, **72**
Mesenteric adenitis, 43
Mesenteric cyst, 26
Mesoblastic nephroma, 51
Metastatic disease, 95
    abdominal, 27
    hepatic, 52
    pulmonary, 11, 24
    spinal involvement, 83
MLCN. *See* Multilocular cystic nephroma
Mucopolysaccharidoses, 81

Multicystic dysplastic kidney, 31, **44**, 46
Multilocular cystic nephroma, **46**
Multiple sclerosis (MS), 80

N
Nasal polyp, 74
Navicular bone, normal, 90
Necrotizing enterocolitis (NEC), **42**
Nephroblastomatosis, **47**, 57
Nephrolithiasis, **55**
Nephroma
    mesoblastic, 51
    multilocular cystic, **46**
Neurenteric cyst, 23
Neuroblastoma, **7**, 35, 51, 66
    metastases, 95
        abdominal, 27
        spinal, 83
Neurofibroma, 7
Newborn
    pneumonia in, 5
    transient tachypnea of, 5
Nonossifying fibroma (NOF), **97**

O
Obstructive uropathy, **57**
OI. *See* Osteogenesis imperfecta
Omega epiglottis, 9
Omental infarction, **45**
Osteogenesis imperfecta, 92, **96**
Osteoid osteoma, 88, **98**
Osteomyelitis, 84, 85, 86, 90, 95, 98
Osteosarcoma, **84**, 94
    telangiectatic, 93
Ovarian cyst, hemorrhagic, 64
Ovarian teratoma, **65**
Ovarian torsion, **64**
Ovarian tumor, 64, 65
    cystic, 62

P
Pancreas, annular, 33
Pancreatic ductal system, anomalies, 50
Pancreatitis
    acute, **50**
    traumatic, 50
Papillomatosis, **24**
    laryngotracheal, 22
Pericardial effusion, 21
Periventricular leukomalacia, 76
Perthes disease. *See* Legg-Calvé-Perthes disease
PIE. *See* Pulmonary interstitial emphysema
Pilocytic astrocytoma, 72
Pneumonia, 15
    cavitary, 8
    community-acquired, 4
    necrotizing, 13

Pneumonia (*continued*)
  neonatal, 5
  round, **11**
Polycystic kidney disease
  autosomal dominant, 59, **60**
  autosomal recessive, **59**
Polyp, nasal, 74
Porencephaly, 77
Posterior reversible encephalopathy syndrome, 76, 80
Posterior urethral valves, **30**
Postprandial state, 53
Pseudocoarctation, 20
Pulmonary adenomatous malformation, congenital, 8, **13**
Pulmonary artery
  congenital absence of, **14**
  hypoplasia/agenesis, 16
Pulmonary atresia with intact ventricular septum, 21
Pulmonary interstitial emphysema, **18**
Pulmonary metastases, 11, 24
Pulmonary sequestration, 2, **3**
Pulmonary sling, **19**
Pyelonephritis, 56
Pyloric stenosis, hypertrophic, **33**, **39**
Pylorospasm, 39

R
Rathke cleft cyst, 73
Renal cysts, simple, 60
Renal dysplasia, cystic, 59
Renal infarction, 57
Rhabdomyosarcoma, **34**, 74
  pulmonary metastases, 11
Rickets, **82**, 96

S
Salter-Harris fracture(s), 100
  type I, **100**
Scheuermann disease, 83
Schizencephaly, **77**
Schwachman-Diamond syndrome, 25
Scimitar syndrome, **2**
SDD. *See* Surfactant deficiency disease
Septic arthritis, 86
Septo-optic dysplasia, 77
Shoulder, normal, 100
Shunt catheter. *See* Ventriculoperitoneal shunt catheter
Sickle cell disease, acute chest syndrome in, **4**
Slipped capital femoral epiphysis, 89, **91**
SOD. *See* Septo-optic dysplasia
Spinal neoplasm, 83
Steeple sign, 9
Steroid therapy, 25
Stress fracture

of hip, 98
  tibial, **88**
Sturge-Weber syndrome, 68
Subdural hematoma, 67
Supracondylar fracture, **87**
Surfactant deficiency disease, partially treated, 18
Swyer-James syndrome, 14, **16**
Syphilis, 82

T
Telangiectatic osteosarcoma, 93
Testicular torsion, **63**
Thanatophoric dysplasia, **81**
Thyroglossal duct cyst, 71
Thyroid, lingual, **71**
Tibial stress fracture, **88**
Toddler fracture, **86**
Tonsil, lingual, enlarged, 71
TORCH, sequela, 70
Toxic synovitis, 86, 99
Transient tachypnea of newborn, 5
Tuberculosis, **12**
Tuberous sclerosis, 60, **70**
Tumor(s). *See also specific tumor*
  giant cell, 85
  neural, 7
  ovarian, 64, 65
    cystic, 62
  Wilms. *See* Wilms tumor

U
Ureteral duplication, complete, with upper pole ureterocele, **54**
Ureteropelvic junction (UPJ) obstruction, **31**
Ureterovesical junction (UVJ) obstruction, 30, 31

V
VACTERL association, **1**
Vein of Galen malformation, **78**
Venous malformation, abdominal, 61
Ventriculoperitoneal shunt catheter
  abandoned, 79
  disrupted, **79**
  pseudo-disruption, 79
Vesicoureteral reflux (VUR), 30, **58**
Viral bronchiolitis, **15**

W
"Wandering" duodenum, 41
Wegener's granulomatosis, 22
Wilms tumor, 44, 47, **51**
  cystic, 46
  pulmonary metastases, 11, 24

X
X-linked adrenoleukodystrophy, **76**